DILEMMA IN SURGICAL PRACTICE

PROF. P. SIVALINGAM

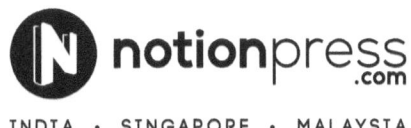

INDIA • SINGAPORE • MALAYSIA

Notion Press

Old No. 38, New No. 6
McNichols Road, Chetpet
Chennai - 600 031

First Published by Notion Press 2020
Copyright © Prof. P. Sivalingam 2020
All Rights Reserved.

ISBN 978-1-64805-715-1

This book has been published with all efforts taken to make the material error-free after the consent of the author. However, the author and the publisher do not assume and hereby disclaim any liability to any party for any loss, damage, or disruption caused by errors or omissions, whether such errors or omissions result from negligence, accident, or any other cause.

While every effort has been made to avoid any mistake or omission, this publication is being sold on the condition and understanding that neither the author nor the publishers or printers would be liable in any manner to any person by reason of any mistake or omission in this publication or for any action taken or omitted to be taken or advice rendered or accepted on the basis of this work. For any defect in printing or binding the publishers will be liable only to replace the defective copy by another copy of this work then available.

CONTENTS

Preface — 5
1. As a House Surgeon. — 7
2. Casualty Medical Officer. — 9
3. Trauma. — 12
4. Injury Due to Assault. — 18
5. Head Injury. — 22
6. Fire in Cracker Shop. — 25
7. Surgery for Spleen. — 27
8. Tracheostomy. — 30
9. Tetanus. — 32
10. Intractable Ascites Due to Cirrhosis Liver. — 36
11. Hernia. — 39
12. Incisional Hernia. — 47
13. Breast. — 51
14. Thyroid Surgery. — 53
15. Complications of Spinal Anaesthesia. — 55
16. Urgent Call for Bleeding. — 57
17. Urinary Bladder and Urethra. — 60
18. Tumour Testis. — 63
19. Obstetric and Gynace Cases. — 65
20. Acute Appendicitis. — 68
21. Gall Bladder Surgery. — 76
22. Bowel Perforations. — 79

23. Bowel Obstruction.	88
24. Anal Problems.	100
25. Colonic Pathology.	112
26. Rectal Conditions.	116
27. Other Rare Conditions.	126
28. Honour in My Professional Career.	134
Annexure	*137*

PREFACE

"Commit yourself to the person who comes seeking help'.

"If you tell the truth you do not have to remember anything".

I am fortunate to be in the teaching side for 31 years and one and half years in district head quarter hospital. I just recollected my certain interesting cases where had dilemma in diagnosis or management during my surgical practice over more than 40 years.

Medical profession is different. The more cases you see the more knowledge you gain, at least one point you learn in each critically ill patients. In those days general surgeons were doing all surgical cases including gynaec, ortho and even cardio thoracic and neuro cases. In those days in southern part of Tamil Nadu, the great surgeon Dr.P.Vadamalayan M.B; B.S; in 1940 to 1970 proved himself capable of doing all surgeries. Now this could not be because specialities have developed and the surgeons are limited in their field. It is said general surgeons are those know a little about all fields where as a specialty people know more about a little field.

I qualified to be a general surgeon in 1970, the period we depend on the clinical experiences in making diagnosis and treating the patients. If any doubt about the diagnosis, repeated examinations were made in a day particularly in emergency cases. Now the diagnosis is made with modern equipments like Endoscopes, Abdominal Scan, C.T, MRI, PET scan and more. During my later half my practice, after my training in colorectal surgery in U.K, I had the help from modern investigating equipments. Days may come when the diagnosis may be made without touching the patient and surgery may be done without the human touch.

Still I remember during my house surgeon days and PG period, we give open ether for minor cases like drainage of pus, suture of wounds. Spinal anaesthesia was given by surgical side assistants and PG students. Reusable IV sets, syringes and needles were sterilized in boiling water. Now they are available as disposable pre sterilised packets. The senior people who read this book on "Dilemma in Surgical Practice" will recollect how they faced the problematic cases and how they managed them. Their technique may not be in scientific way in the modern era, but they saved more patients. The success of surgery is widely helped by the advancements, particularly in anaesthesia and the new instruments. Surgery is never static; *it changes to find out some new techniques to improve the quality of outcome.*

In spite of advanced technology, skill full hands and brilliant mind, we have our own human limitations. The young surgeons who read this book will appreciate how the surgeons struggled to treat the patient. Some of the interesting cases which I have come across were discussed which I think may be useful for young surgeons.

Prof. P. SIVALINGAM. MS; MNAMS.

Retired Professor and Head of the Department of Surgery

Madurai medical college Madurai.

Colorectal Surgeon. Govt. Rajaji Hospital Madurai.

80 B, P.T.Rajan Road.BiBi Kulam. Madurai 625002. TamilNadu.

Phone: 0452 2531543 : 2531703.

Email: drpsivalingam@yahoo.com

1. AS A HOUSE SURGEON.

1.1. SUDDEN CHANGE IN PULSE RATE AND BLOOD PRESSURE.

In 1965 when I was doing my house surgeon, during my duty days I used to check the B.P, pulse rate and intake and output chart for all 7 cases in post operative ward at 7 PM and then go to main ward, and other wards and wait in the post operative ward for the assistant rounds. At about 9.30 PM before I go for my dinner I Check the pulse and B.P for all the patients in post operative ward. One of my duty days I checked the B P and pulse rate at 7 P.M and waiting for the assistant rounds. At about 8-30 PM one patient in the post operative ward suddenly complains of abdominal pain and vomiting.

When I examined him, the Pulse rate has increased and B P was low. As phone services are not available on those days in many places, I went to the assistant Dr.Nayak house which was very close to the hospital and informed the condition of the patient. He came with me to the hospital, saw the case and decided to take up the case for surgery immediately. He asked me to get one unit of blood. He operated the Case. It was a care of duodenal ulcer for which vagotomy and gastro jejunostomy was done. The patient survived from stormy post operative period.

1.2. SCABIES INFESTATION IN ALL IMMATES OF THE HOSTEL.

When I was doing house surgeon in Social and Preventive Medicine department, I was posted in Primary sub Centre at Palamedu. One boy of about 10 years of age came to the outpatient clinic for the treatment of Scabies. I asked him whether other family members have lesions like this. He said he is staying in Govt. Hostel in Palamedu. I told that Boy that I will be coming to your hostel that evening and asked to tell the warden. I went to the hostel saw all the inmates there. Almost everybody including the warden had scabies. I told the warden that I will be coming on Saturday morning at 7AM to treat all the inmates of the hostel. One person from

Andhra Pradesh doing PhD in Mahatma Gandhi Rural University was staying with me in Palamedu for one month. I asked him to bring 5 Litres of Benzyl Benzoate from Gandhi Gram Hospital for the treatment of scabies. He brought Benzyl Benzoate. I bought some cheakkai powder and some shaving blades to cut the nails. That Saturday morning myself and that Andhra man went to the hostel. I asked all the students to cut the nails close and to remove the dresses except the underwear. All students took bath with Cheakkai powder particularly the affected area including the genital area. After the body becomes dry I showed them how to apply Benzyl Benzoate throughout the body except the head and face. I asked them to wash all the dresses and bed sheets. I asked them to apply Benzyl Benzoate on Saturday night and Sunday morning and take bath on Monday morning. Next Saturday morning I went to the hostel, I am surprised to see almost all scabies lesions have gone and the students are happy including the warden. With one day visit to the hostel, I have eradicated scabies in 15 students. The Andhra man appreciated my approach to treat the community. I told him it was possible only because you brought benzyl Benzoate.

2. CASUALTY MEDICAL OFFICER.

2.1. AVULSION OF SCALP.

On the previous day of Diwali in1971, I was on duty in the casualty. At about 6 AM one lady accompanied by a male attender came to the casualty covering her head with blood stained cloth. I examined the patient. It was a case of avulsion of the Scalp and it was attached to the Skull in the occipital region only. When I asked how it was happened the patient said she went to rice mill to grind the rice after taking bath and without combing her hairs. The hairs got in the belt of the rice mill machine, immediately the machine was stopped and the rice mill people asked her to go to Government hospital for treatment. I entered the case in the accident register as a medico legal case and admitted her and informed the Police. Next day when I came for the duty the SI of GRH out post Police Station said that the injury is not due to rice mill belt. There was a family quarrel between this lady and her husband, the husband got hold of her hairs and gave a Kick on her Chest and so the avulsion of the scalp has occurred. The husband also has accepted and a case has been booked against him. When he came to the casualty he never opened his mouth so I thought he may be from rice mill or one of her neighbours.

2.2. ALLEGED BULL GORE INJURY.

A man was brought to casualty as Bull gore injury by four people. As I stood up from the chair to see the patient, I heard a lady shouting outside the casualty in the road saying,' "Ada paveekala", you stabbed my husband'. I immediately asked everybody to wait outside and asked the nursing assistant to bring that lady. The lady said she is the wife of that patient, these people stabbed him and brought him here as bull hore injury. I asked the patient what has happened and he narrated the incidence as stab wound. I made prober entry in the accident register as Stab injury, admitted him and informed the police out post. I was told by the nursing assistance that the people who brought the patient to the casualty ran away before the police come to the casualty.

2.3. ALLEGED FALL INTO A WELL.

A patient was referred from Dindugal hospital as fall into the well. As I am not happy with the way the accompanying people behaviour, I asked the patients what has happened. The patient refused to talk with me and only accompanied persons answered my questions. So made entry in the accident register, admitted the patient and informed the Police out post. After two days the police from outpost told me that the person was assaulted with wooden blocks and pushed him into the well and Dindugal Police has registered the case against his two Sons.

These three cases are good examples that when we see any case with injury, it is better to enter in the accident register and inform the police. It is up to the police to investigate the case whether it is assault or accident. Even entry in the accident register will be accepted in the Court as evident in some cases. If you don't enter the case in accident register you may face trouble after words.

2.4. ASTHMA PATIENTS STAY IN THE HOSPITAL VERANDA IN THE NIGHT.

In those days (1971) there was no city Bus service after 10 PM and here is no auto service in Madurai. So the patients have to come to hospital either by cycle rickshaw or by Chaka pulled by horse and that too in a limited area and limited services. So the asthma patients stay in the hospital veranda during December and January months when the asthma attacks are severe in cold conditions. When the asthma attack occurs they get the injection for asthma either aminophyline or Decadron or adrenaline. There are drugs available at those times for asthma. I have gave in standing instruction to the duty nurse to give injection of what the patients want at that particular time because they know which drug will be effective for them, don't make them to wait for the token for the injection and get the token singed later. These people are not financially poor. When they get intolerable asthma symptoms in the night, transport services will not be available in the night so they come to the hospital and sleep and when required they get the injection. Now more medicines are available in tablet form, liquid form and Puff for asthma patients and the transport services are available all the time.

2.5. PAPER ON DOG BITE; PRESENTED IN CLINICAL SOCIETY MEETING.

"If you want to be the best, you have to do things that other people are not willing to do".

For the first time in the history of Govt Rajaji Hospital Clinical Society meeting, from casualty a paper on Dog Bite was presented in 1971. Three months statistics of dog bites were collected from the Casualty. All cases of dog bites were treated only in casualty on those days. So collecting the data was not difficult. Within three months 1330 cases were treated in the casualty during April, May and June 1971. It forms roughly 443 cases for a month and 15 cases per day.

My aims was after presenting in Clinical Society meeting and make update of the paper with the points from the discussion, sent it to Madurai Corporation to take active steps to control the stray dogs in Madurai and reduce the number of incidence of dog bite in Madurai and eradicate the Rabies which is potentially fatal. Positive works make you happy light and refreshed.

3. TRAUMA.

3.1. A GIRL PREPARING FOR ENTRANCE EXAMINATION.

That day was Tamil New Year day. We wanted to go to Meenakshi Amman Temple in the evening at 5.30. Before going to the temple my wife wanted to see a case in Vadamalayan hospital. I was waiting in the car in the hospital. A taxi came with a patient. I helped the hospital servants to transfer the patient from the taxi to the Strercher and asked the reception counter people to inform the doctor immediately about this case. She told me that this case has been referred to you only. I examined the patient in the outpatient examine room. There was evidence of Pelvic Fracture with heavy bleeding from the lacerated wound in the back and thigh. Bladder was characterized and clear urine was let out, which exclude bladder injury. lV drip was started in one arum and asked the duly doctor to start blood in the other arm. l gave instruction to take Bed X Ray Pelvis, antibiotics and sedation. As it may take one hour to resuscitate the patient we went to temple and returned. The patient was reviewed in the operation theatre. There was lacerated wound in the back, gluteal region and the perineum. The wounds were cleaned and dressed to prevent further bleeding.

The Pelvic fracture was seen by the orthopaedic surgeon and advised conservative treatment. After 2 days when the patient was stable defunct ion colostomy was done to prevent wound contamination with faeces. She was treated in the hospital for 6 weeks after the wound healed reasonably, she was discharged with colostomy. I made her as a member of Ostomy Association Madurai chapter and she attended annual meeting of the association. She wanted the colostomy to be closed. I told her if you are able to do Squatting Position as you sit during defecation I will close the colostomy and asked her to do that exercise daily and come after 2 months. Every time the she comes to me with the hopeful that I will close the colostomy at that time and finally after 6 months the colostomy was closed when I am satisfied with her squatting position. I was very particular that she must be able to sit in Squatting position otherwise she has to pass motion in standing position which will be an embracing situation for a girl of 18 years of age.

3.2. SPLENIC INJURY IN PREGNANCY (LOURDU MARY).

The Female patient Lourdu Mary was admitted in Trauma ward for run over by a lorry in evening duty hours. I came for duty at 8 PM and this case was handed over as said to have run over by a lorry but she is stable and X-ray's were normal said Dr.Nagaian, the senior assistant under whom I have worked as PG. When I examined her half an hour after he left, the patient had tachycardia and low blood pressure. Dr.Nagaian never writes the pulse rate in the case sheet without himself counted. Patient complains of pain in the chest and abdomen. She told us she is pregnant. X-ray showed multiple fractures of the Ribs on the left side with haemo- pneumothorax. When I asked the radiographer whether Dr.Nagaian seen this X-ray. He said no body has seen this X-ray but the house surgeon has shown some X ray to him but I did not realize that he has taken by mistake another X ray. I immediately started the treatment. Left intercostals drainage was done under local. Arrangements were made for Blood transfusion, urinary bladder catheterisation was done, nasal 02 started. I suspected injury of the spleen. I liked to have gynaecologist opinion and so the duty doctor was called. She saw the case and said she will call the senior person. After some time, my classmate Dr.Sivakamasundari came. She said at present there is no evidence of rupture of uterus and the pregnancy is normal. She told me if you are taking up this case for surgery please look the uterus and if necessary call us. The general condition of the patient has not improved with treatment. I told the anaesthetist I will take all the responsibility and give anaesthesia for this patient. On laparotomy the Spleen was found lacerated with bleeding. Splenectomy was done. The uterus and other viscera were found normal. I saw the patient next-day during my night rounds. Three days later I saw her.

She was restless, severely dehydrated and scanty urine out put through the catheter. When I asked the nurse how much fluids was given in the day time. She said IV fluids were stopped and the patient is not taking anything orally. I started 1V fluids and I was with the patient till 2 litres of fluids were over and the output of 200 cc and asked the nurse to continue another 1.5 litres till the morning. Next day the patient expelled dead foetus. Later she was transferred to post operative ward and died after 2 days with multi organ failure. I could not do anything in the post operative ward because she belongs to some other unite.

3.3. ROAD TRAFIC ACCIDENT. FEMORAL ARTERY SPASM.

An electrical Engineer son Syed was admitted in trauma ward for injuries due to bus accident. There was extensive lacerated wound in the right thigh, exposing the femoral vessels and nerves. The femoral artery was in severe spasm with vascular impediment. Lignocaine was infiltrated around the femoral artery. Left side Lumbar Sympathetic nerve Block was done by the anaesthetist Dr.Lakshmi. The femoral artery spasm slowly relieved and femoral artery pulsation could be seen. The wound debridement was done and left opens for delayed primary suture. The patient was resuscitated with blood and IV fluids and antibiotics. On the 4th day Femoral artery Thrormpectomy was done by the cardiothoracic surgeon. The thigh wounds are managed with partial suturing and later Skin grafting and the patient was discharged with residual foot drop right side.

3.4. SUPRA CONDYLAR FRACTURE WITH BRACHIAL ARTERY SPASM.

On those days some of uncomplicated cases of fractures, the DAS will do the reduction of the fracture under sedation or short GA. After I passed M.S. general surgery in1970 I will be seeing all emergency surgeries done by the DAS all the days up to 1974. I requested all duty anaesthetists to inform me whenever any emergency surgery to be done by DAS. They inform the time of emergency surgery by phone even after my marriage. I carefully see how the senior DAS are doing surgery and how my colleague are struggling to manage the case. One case of supra condylar fracture emergency reduction was done under short GA because of feeble pulse of radial artery on that side. After reduction even that feeble pulse was not palpable. Dr.Rajappa who was an ex military service man, exposed the Brachial artery which was with severe spasm and looked like a thread. By anatomical situation, I told him that tread like structure is the brachial artery. As I have worked in Anatomy department for 2 years before I join PG course I was confident in localising the brachial artery'. Papavarin liquid was instilled over the brachial artery and later Lignocaine was instilled for vasodilatation. As the spasm still continued I asked the anaesthetist Dr.Padma lakshmi, who worked with me in Tirunelveli medical College to give supra clavicular Brachial Block to relieve the spasm. She said so far I have not given supra clavicular block. I told her give it as the first case and she succeeded in giving the block and Brachial artery Pulsation slowly regained and the pulsation of the brachial artery and radial artery restored. The fracture was reduced and now the Radial Pulse was palpable after reduction of the Fracture and POP was applied. We are all happy that vascular ischemia of the upper limb was prevented and its Complication of Volkmann ischemic contracture was prevented.

3.5. ROAD TRAFFIC ACCIDENT. PARA DUODENAL COLLECTION.

A Lady from Coimbatore was driving a car to Madurai met with an accident. She was admitted in some other hospital in Madurai and I was asked to see her. The patient was related to a doctor couple. There was no external injury. She had fracture Femur and Humerus on the left side. Upper Abdominal tenderness present but no muscle guarding and X ray abdomen there was no gas under the diaphragm. The patient was quite stable and so as far as the abdominal injury, it was decided to treat conservatively as there is no definite indication for surgery. The fractures were treated by orthopaedic surgeon. On the 3rd day of admission she had vomiting and a feeling of abdominal distension. Abdominal ultra sonogram showed collection in the Para duodenal region and head of the pancreas. Under ultra sonic guidance aspiration of clear fluid was done. The vomiting and feeling of abdominal distension had subsided. Aspiration had been repeated after one week and after ten days of second aspiration. The patient was discharged and went home. Later I was told she delivered twins at Coimbatore.

3.6. ROAD TRAFFIC ACCIDENT – BILATERAL THORACOTOMY DONE.

A male patient was admitted for run over Chest by a car. The patient had lacerated wound over the left side of the chest and haemopneumothorax in the right side with fracture Ribs on both sides. Both sides intercostals drainage was done. There were air leaks in both sides. So it was decided to take up the case to the theatre. First the left side of the chest was opened and the lung, injury was sutured. The right side of the chest was opened and the injured lung was sutured and the chest wounds were closed with ICD in both sides. The surgery was over by 3.30 PM and I checked whether ICD were functioning. The anaesthetist Dr.Kanagaraj said hats off to you, sir, usually the surgeons leave the theatre after the surgery, but you are in side till the patient recover from anaesthesia and cheek the ICD. Check X ray chest showed both ICD tubes were in correct position. The Cardiothoracic surgeon Dr.GowriSankar came for night rounds and I showed the case to him. He examined the patient and saw the check X-ray and asked me to remove one ICD in next day morning and asked which side I am going to remove. I told him I will remove the tube on the right side. He said he will see the case next day during morning rounds with check X-ray.

3.7. HAEMOPERICARDIUM WITH CARDIAC TAMPONADE.

A leading doctor from Karaikudi was admitted in accident ward for Road traffic accident while travelling in a car. The driver of the car was also had injury. We were informed before hand and we were waiting for their arrival. Totally three people were injured including the doctor. When I went to examine her she said I am alright you first see the driver and the other person. The other person had fracture of Humerus and some abrasions. The driver had chest injuries with haemo pneumothorax and lCD was done. Now I came to see the doctor. She said she has some compressing pain in the chest. She become dyspneic and the neck vein become distended. The patient was shifted to X ray room as I suspected Cardiac tampenade due to pericardial blood collection. The patient cannot sit properly for X-ray chest. I was with the patients in the X ray room and the patient died in the X-ray table. Next day I went to forensic department to know the autopsy report. They said there was haemopericardium which was the cause of death. If I have taken X-ray Chest immediately after admission there would have been minimal Collection of blood in the Pericardium and we would have vigorous monitoring. But she asked me to see the driver and the other person. It was a bad day for me that a leading doctor died is my duty time.

3.8. FALL FROM A COCONUT TREE.

A case was admitted from casualty as fall from a coconut tree. When I asked the accompanying persons what happened they said he has fallen from a coconut tree. As the condition of the patient was serious, I asked the post graduate trainee to start the drip and cortisone injection. When one bottle of I.V. fluid was over the patient developed pulmonary oedema and within half an hour he died. I explained the condition of the patient to the relatives; one of them said what you can do sir he fell into the well from the coconut tree. We tried to bring him up from the well and two times he slipped from our hands and again fell into well. With great difficulty we brought him out of well. When I asked them if he has fallen into the well how the dresses are dry. We changed the dresses in the house before we come to the hospital. So essentially it is a case of drowning. The treatment is different for drowning. The patient was admitted from casualty as fall from coconut tree and the accompanying persons were also said the same and the condition of the patient is bad, the patient was treated as fall from a height. I never suspected drowning because the dresses of the patient were not wet.

3.9. ELECTRIC INJURY.

A 25 years male was admitted with electric burns in both upper limbs. On examination the evidence of point of entry in left axilla, the points of exists was in the right arm with extensive damage. On the 5th day of admission as I was going for routine ward rounds before going to operation theatre, I saw this patient had evidence of bleeding in left axilla. I examined the wound. The bleeding was from left brachial artery. With the available instruments the brachial artery was ligated and the bleeding stopped. This was done at 8:15AM and I went to the operation theatre 15 minutes late. Others were waiting for me to start the case. People thought I will say sorry for coming late to the operation theatre but I scolded the main ward P.G. and house surgeons for not seeing the patient in the ward before coming to the operation theatre. They said they saw the main ward patients but not gone to where the septic cases were kept.

I told them why I have come late. One week later gangrene on the right forearm developed due infection. So the patient was posted for above elbow amputation. When the surgeon ligated the brachial artery, the anaesthetist said stop the surgery, Peripheral pulse could not be palpable, Let me do something for that. But the auxiliary artery pulsations are seen on the side where we are operating. Then only I recollected the incidence of brachial artery ligation on the left side and told him. Then the anaesthetist permitted to precede the surgery. Now my doubt was whether the anaesthetist recorded the pulse on the left side, before giving anaesthesia.

4. INJURY DUE TO ASSAULT.

4.1. MULTIPLE CUT INJURY SCALP.

A patient was admitted for multiple scalp injuries due to assault with sharp weapon. The patient was conscious and there was excessive bleeding from the scalp wounds. The patient was rushed to the operation theatre and general anaesthesia was given. The scalp was shaved by the barber and simultaneously all the wounds are explored for bone involvement. Fortunately there was no bony and X Ray skull was normal. All the wounds in the scalp were sutured. Documentation we made only made after the treatment. The patient was discharged after suture removal.

4.2. ARURAL CUT IN THE CENTER OF THE SCALP.

The patient Mr. Muniyandi was admitted in our ward for Aruval cut injury scalp. Before opening the trauma ward in madurai all the patients were admitted in general surgical wards in the admitting unit. That day we had four emergency operations in the night and we were coming out from operation theatre at 3.30 AM and the patient just coming to the ward from casualty. I asked PG to see the X ray of the Skull for fracture and if there is no fracture then suture the scalp wound. I came to the ward at 5 AM and saw the X-ray which showed depressed fracture in the parietal bone close to midline. Immediately I sent the memo to the duty assistant surgeon in neurosurgery department (Dr.Balakrishnan). He wrote in the case sheet that the depressed fracture would have been elevated yesterday itself and as the wound was sutured and as such there is no neurological defect the case can be observed. When I examined the patient during morning rounds at 9am he developed hemiplegia. Now I sent memo to the neuro surgery assistant and I continued the ward rounds. Dr.M.N. called me and asked me tell me frankly did you see the X-ray before suturing the wound. I said no but I asked the PG to see the X-ray before suturing the wound. I saw the X-ray at 5am. He said because you have missed the depressed fracture, you do the elevation in our neuro theatre with the help of Dr.Balakrishnan, the neuro assistant and treat the case in your ward. I did the elevation of depressed fracture of frontal bone with great care to avoid injury to the superior saggital sinus. Since some broken pieces were loose in certain areas they were removed, the edges of the frontal bone were nipped out gel form applied and the scalp wound was sutured. Post operatively the patient was treated in our main ward. The patient had recovered from hemiplegia. He was discharged after 2 weeks. The only complication he had was stricture urethra due do prolonged use of catheter and infection which was treated by urethral dilatation. Each time when he comes for dilatation I call the students to see brain pulsations due to the bone defect.

4.3. STAB INJURY IN A TWO YEARS CHILD.

A Child was brought to the trauma ward with gangrenous small intestine protruding throw a small stab wound in the abdominal wall. The child was rushed to the operation theatre and under general anaesthesia the wound was explored. A small defect of 2 CM was noted through which the small intestine was protruding and 5 CM of the bowel was gangrene. The gangrenous part is excised and end to end anatomises was done. There was no other Injury and the abdomen was closed. The resuscitation of the child was done by one of the anaesthetist and the other man gave anaesthesia. Without the help of the anaesthetist doctors Aziz and Murugadoss, the child could not been saved. In this case the spirit of team work has helped.

4.4. STAB INJURY RIGHT LOIN.

One patient was admitted for stab wound in the loin. He has taken alcohol and full meal in the night one hour before the incidence. I wanted to explore the wound under local and if necessary exploratory laparotomy. The duty anaesthetist Dr Krishnan said we wait for 4 hours as he has taken full meals. So after 4 hours the wound was explored under local anaesthesia. The wound had communication will the peritoneal cavity. So it was decided to do exploratory laparotomy to find out any injury to the internal organ. During intubation of endotracheal tube patient vomited briyani and had persistent retching and vomiting. So it was decided to give spinal anaesthesia in sitting position. Repeated throat suction was applied to suck out briyani and the secretions from the respiratory tract. There was no internal organ injury. The peritoneal defect was closed and the abdomen was closed in layers.

4.5. STAB INJURY RIGHT HYPOCHONDRIUM.

A political party worker Mr.MuthuKnishnan said to have been stabbed while he was reading news paper in the veranda of his house, on the right side of epigastrium. He was rushed to the casualty and got admitted in accident ward. On examination there was only one injury of about 5cm length in the epigastrium more on the right side, and blood was pouring out from the wound. I suspected liver injury. By the time more party workers came to the accident ward. I told to one of the leaders of the party that he may need 6 to 7 units of blood and please make arrangement to donate the blood; I will let you know the blood group of the patient within a short period. The patient was rushed to the operation theatre. When I asked the patient who had stabbed he said I know but I will not say now. Under anaesthesia shaving of the abdomen and other skin preparations were done by the post graduate while I was ready with operation dress. The abdomen was opened. There was a large collection of blood in the peritoneal cavity which was removed by suction. There was a penetrating wound in the right lobe of the liver and when a probe was passed through the injury site of the liver, the probe went up to the Porta hepatica. So the lesser sac was opened and the bleeding from the hepatic artery was arrested by Pringles' technique between the thumb and index finger. The hepatic artery was ligated. Even after ligation of the hepatic artery there was venous bleeding and on careful examination it was from the Inferior Venae Cava. The bleeding was controlled by packing the area and cardiothoracic surgeon was called. The patient died before cardiothoracic surgeon came. The party workers donated 8 units of blood and all 8 units are used for the patient. I explained the situation to the party workers and the death was declared after shifting the patient to the ward.

Next day I went to Forensic department at about I.30 PM, I heard Dr.Sempon David saying that it is how the recording must be done, at that time I entered his room and on seeing me he said 'see the Devil has come' I told him about what had happened to the patient Muthuknishnan. He said we are discussing about that case only and I told the assistance it is how the recording must be done. The Post-mortem findings are all exactly what you have described. The injury to Inferior venae cava was found which was not closed. I explained the situation why Inferior venae cava was not sutured. After some months Dr.Sempon David and myself attended the court regarding this case.

4.6. STAB INJURY IN THE RIGHT SIDE OF THE NECK.

A patient was admitted with penetrating wound in the lower part of the neck on the right side. Venous bleeding from the wound was present. Under local the wound was explored and the cut ends of the external Jugular vein were located and ligated and the wound was sutured. The patient had a bout of cough and bleeding occurred from the wound. The patient was taken to the operation theatre and under general anaesthesia the wound was examined. Injury was made cut at the junction of internal jugular vein and the Subclavian Vein. My Chief Dr. Kalidoss and Cardiothoracic surgeon Dr.Andappan were called. The injured site in internal jugular vein was sutured by Dr.Andappan. Five units of A Group Blood were donated by the relatives. Patient died after 2 days.

5. HEAD INJURY.

5.1. BUS ACCIDENT TO A BOY OF 8 YEARS.

A boy of 8 years was brought by his father for the treatment of injury due to Bus accident. I entered in Accident register and I admitted the patient. The father of the patient is a worker in T.V.S. Company said as the boy is otherwise normal, I don't want admission. With half mind I cancelled the admission and treated the boy as outpatient and I have not informed the Police. But I entered the father's statement in the Accident register. Two days later the boy was brought to the casualty with evidence of cerebral compression. The duty casualty medical office admitted the boy after entering in Accident register in the page where I have written two days back and the boy died on that day. After 2 days the father has sent a letter to the Dean of Govt. Rajaji hospital, describing the events and asked for the death certificate. The Dean Dr.Kabir called me and asked about the incidence. I showed him the Accident register where I have mentioned that the father did not want admission and so the admission was cancelled and treated as outpatient. The father also had written the same thing in the letter. Dr.Kabir said you are all Bandits in your field, though there was no fault on your side, you might have admitted. From that incidence on wards when I think that particular patient needs admission I just write in the OP ticket admit.

If the patient says that he has to inform his family members I tell them that this signature is valid up to 12 midnight. So you can get admitted at any time before 12 mid night today, and I never cancel admission and never prescribe any medicine.

5.2. OCCIPITAL HAEMATOMA.

When I went for accident wand duty in the morning one patient was handed over to me as lumbar spine fracture. After taking over at 7 AM, I made detailed ward rounds. The patient, who was told as fracture lumbar spine, had occipital haematoma with decerebrated rigidity with shallow respiration. Pupils could not be seen as the patient had bilateral blindness. The patient died within 30 minutes. The trend has come in accident ward, the duty general surgeon sees only general surgery cases and they don't see other cases like ortho or Cardio thoracic cases and neuro cases. They must see all the cases who were admitted in accident ward.

I was told by one cardio thoracic surgeon that he was called to see a case in the night. When he came, the duty Assistant on duty was sleeping. The Thoracic surgeon saw the case. The patient needed I.C.D. so called the duty doctor to do ICD. The duty assistant surgeon told him that it is a thoracic case and you do the ICD. I do not know how to put inter costal drain. When the Thoracic surgeon was doing inter costal drain, the duly assistant surgeon went for sleep. I told the thoracic surgeon, if anybody says like that to me, I will tell them I will teach you how to put inter costal drain; you please wash up and come.

Like this another incidence happened to me. My assistance was called from trauma ward to see a case. Dr. Mustafa saw the case and he advised immediate colostomy with Todd's Bridge and has written in the case sheet itself. The duty assistance has told him that he did not know how to do Colostomy with Todd's Bridge and so you do it. Dr. Mustafa came back to colorectal op and said what has happened in the accident ward. I told Dr. Mustafa, ask the duty assistant in the accident ward to give it in writing that he did not know how to do colostomy with Todd's Bridge then I myself teach him how to do, because that assistant had worked with me for some time. Now the assistant told Dr. Mustafa that he will do the case and requested Dr Mustafa to assist him. That should be the attitude for the youngsters. When they do not know one technique they can have the help of others but they should not say ' I do not know and so you do it '.

5.3. EMERGENCY BURR HOLE.

The neuro PG Dr Suresh told me that he is going to do **Burr hole** for a case from accident ward at 9 AM on that day. After clearing the op cases which came for suturing of the wounds I started ward rounds at about 9-30 am. When examined one head injury case, he had Brady cardia and unequal pupils and disorientation. The neurosurgeon Dr.M.Natarajan who made rounds in the accident ward at 8.30AM has written as patient is conscious, pupils are equal reacting to light and Pulse rate as 72. So the cerebral Compression could have occurred after 8.30AM. Now this patient needs immediate surgery. I sent my PG to the emergency operation theatre and to tell Dr. Suresh that an emergency Burr hole is coming now and not to start the first case. If he has already started the case, ask the nurse to keep another table ready for Burr hole. Fortunately the first care was not started.

5.4. RECARDING THE BLOOD PRESSURE AND PULSE FOR A DEAD BODY.

I was in trauma ward day duty for 3 months continuously in 1975. One house surgeon was coming to trauma ward during my duty time. He will do some works when I asked him to do. One day he had regular trauma ward duty for 24 hours in the accident ward. That night the duty assistant asked him to record hourly Blood Pressure and half hourly pulse rate for evaluation of a patient form further treatment. He was doing the recording of the pulse and B.P. very sincerely even the B.P and pulse are not recordable and he has not informed the duty doctor about this.

The duty assistant saw the case at 5 AM and he noticed the pulse and blood pressure are not recordable. He asked the house surgeon from what time the B P and Pulse rates are not recordable. He showed the case sheet and said from I AM. The duty surgeon asked him why he has not informed him, he said you asked me to record hourly B.P and half hourly Pulse rate which I have done. You have not told me to inform you when there is change in B.P. and Pulse rate. In the morning when I came for the duty at 7AM the duty doctor asked me as a first question, what you think about that house surgeon. I told him that he will do sincerely whatever we ask him to do and don't expect anything more from him. The D.A.S said you have judged the person correctly, I asked him to record hourly B.P. and half hourly Pulse rate and he was doing that from 1 AM in a dead body. 'The first principle of true teaching is that nothing can be taught'.

6. FIRE IN CRACKER SHOP.

One Sunday I was on duty is accident ward. One patient came to the casualty with blast injury 12. 30 AM and admitted in accident ward. I asked him how it has occurred. He said there was fire in a cracker shop at about 8 PM in Theni. More people are affected and they are waiting for the transport. I came by lorry as I was alone. He is not sure about the number of deaths. I assessed the nature of the injury and asked the P.G. to treat the case and went to the ward for the preparation for treatment for the coming patients as the patient said about 20-30 patients may come for treatment. I informed the Dean, R.M.O and the nursing superintendent. R.M.O. came and said he will send house surgeons for help. If I relay on too much people I increase the chances of being disappointed so I told him I can manage with our team. I need 5 or 6 stretchers and some wheel Chairs for transporting the patients and ten hospital workers. The Nursing Superintendent asked the duty head nurse to mobilize the hospital workers. I prepared the list of medicines required, like injections Pethedine, Compose, Tetanus Toxoid and tetracycline and sent the list to the Pharmacist. Once the patients came, body bath was given to them in SOT and Tetanus Toxoid, Tetracycline and Sedation were given. The patients who needed only dressing were sent the ward where one nurse was made in charge. Those patients who needed suturing of the wound, suture was done as they were in the Stretchers. Two P.G. are debuted to write the case sheets. Two Senior House surgeons are asked to write the case sheets, send the blood for investigations and start the primary resuscitation treatment for those in serious condition. By 5 AM all the 40 patients are treated. We have seen all the cases again and sent to the ward. Only two cases needed further evaluation. I phoned up to Dr Kalidoss and informed about the cases and asked him to come to see the two cases for medico legal purposes. I requested the Dean to arrange for a separate ward for these patients. He made arrangements in X-ray Block 2nd floor as a separate ward for these patients and separate nurses were posted.All these cases except the two patients, who need further treatment in accident word, were transferred to the separate ward before I leave accident ward. Now the patient's relations can see them will out affecting the regular ward works. As I expected the minister came to the hospital at 10 AM followed by so many VIPs were coming to see the patients.

I left Chennai on the post admission day night and when I saw the newspaper in the morning at Chennai it was published all the patients were treated by accident-ward medical office(by name) whose duty starts at 7 Am only where as the patients were admitted in the midnight and our unit team treated all the cases. Any how our team has done a good job and finished the treatments to all the cases before 5 AM. This was the only day I gave morning tea to our team in my life time as an appreciation of their hard works.

7. SURGERY FOR SPLEEN.

7.1. FALL FROM A WALL.

A 10 years old boy was referred to Vadamalayan hospital by the local doctor in Arupukottai for consultation on Sunday at about I I AM. The patient was examined by my wife Dr.Balasaraswathi and informed me. I saw him at about 12-30 PM. He had injury due to wall collapse while playing in a newly constructed wall. On examination there were aberrations over the left hypochondrium and there was tachycardia low B. P and the patient looked pale. There was tenderness in the upper abdomen more in the left hypochondrium. I suspected injury to the spleen. X-ray chest and abdomen were normal and no fracture of ribs. The mother only had come. I told her he needs immediate surgery and may be expensive. If you want to go to Govt. Hospital I will give you a letter. She said I want you to operate; I will go to my village and bring money and his father. I told her to go to Arupukottai and come back it may take at least 3 hours but the boy needs immediate surgery. She said you do the surgery I will come as early as possible. I verified her address and took the risk of operating the patient without attenders. The spleen was found shattered and so Splenectomy was done. The patient went home without any complication. The mother believed me and the condition of the patient was critical and delay in surgery may lead to death so I took calculated risk in operating without the attenders. By taking risk you are going to lose less. But not taking it you are going to lose more, in medical profession, the life of the patient.

7.2. SUPRA CONDYLAR FRACTURE HUMERUS WITH SPLENIC INJURY.

A case of Supra condylar fracture of left humerus due to car accident was transferred to orthopaedic ward from accident ward. In the evening the orthopaedic PG. Dr. Akbar pasha, who was my classmate, came to me and said he suspects injury to the spleen in a case of supra condylar fracture. I saw the case, it was spleenic injury. The patient was taken up for surgery at 6 PM. In the operation theatre I was discussing with the postgraduates that in Spleenic injury, the abdomen is opened with light anaesthesia without muscle relaxant. Because the abdominal muscle guarding will act like a tampenade effect and the bleeding is controlled to some extent, if the relaxant is given beforehand this tampenade effect will go off and bleeding will occur in the peritoneal cavity. When you are about to open the peritoneum, the anaesthetist must give the muscle relaxant. While opening the abdomen I told the anaesthetist to give muscle relaxant and he gave it. Unfortunately the electricity went off and the suction would not be used. With the help of torch light I put my hand into the spleenic bed and removed the Spleen which was just floating in the peritoneal cavity and packed the spleenic bed with the abdominal pads, waited for some time and removed the pads and got the Spleenic pedicle and ligated. The blood from the peritoneal cavity was removed by the abdominal pads and peritoneal wash was given with 1.5 litres of normal Saline before closing the abdomen. The abdomen was closed with a corrugators rubber drain. The whole surgery was done with torch light only. Once I finished the surgery, the anaesthetist said you have done your job, but how I am going to extubate without suction. I said wait for some time, you will get electricity supply. Let us think of good things and that will occur automatically. After five minutes the power supply restored and extubation was done without any problems and the patient was shifted from the operation table.

7.3. SPLENECTOMY WITH NEPHRECTOMY.

A twelve years boy Muthuraman was admitted in Trauma ward with history of fall from Palmarah tree. There was lacerated injury in the left side of the chest with the Lung exposed and upper abdomen. The relatives said he passed blood stained urine. So bladder was catheterized and few CC of blood stained urine was let out. After optimal resuscitation the patient was taken up for surgery. Thoraco abdominal incision was made on the left side. The foreign bodies in the lung and wound were removed, saline was given the lung injury was sutured. The spleen was floating in the abdomen and the spleen was removed. The spleenic pedicle was ligated. When the Kidneys are examined right kidney was found normal. Left Kidney was completely lacerated and it has to be removed. The diaphragm was sutured. The thoraco abdominal wound was closed with

I.C.D and abdominal drain. On the 3rd Post operative period the patient become breathlessness.

X-ray Chest suggested diaphragmatic hernia. The diaphragmatic hernia was operated by thoracic surgeon Dr. Andappan. The diaphragmatic sutures were given way and the diaphragm was re sutured. The patient developed incision hernia and osteomyelitis of the rib. This case was presented combined with cardiothoracic department in the Clinical Society meeting.

7.4. SPLENECTOMY FOR CONGENITAL SPHEROCYTOSIS.

Splenectomy was done for congenital Spherocytosis. Technically it was simple and the surgery was over within one hour. But there was some problems in recovery from anaesthesia. The chief anaesthetist Dr.Viswanathan, neuro Physician Dr.Sivakumar and the Cardiologist Dr. Srinivasan were called for second opinion and their advices were carried out. The patient had not recovered from anaesthesia and died on the table. Once I finished the surgery I showed the Spleen to the attenders and told them the patient will come out within another 10 minutes. Once the patient died I told the attenders about the death. I told the hospital staff not to collect money for me. But Collect money for other doctors and give it to them. I arranged the Ambulance from Vadamalayan hospital for the transport of the body and the advance money paid by them is adjusted with the theatre expenses. After 15 days the patient's son came and thanked me for providing Ambulance service. After this incidence I show the operated specimen to the attenders only after the patient had recovered from anaesthesia or if done under spinal after the patient was shifted to the stretcher from the operation table.

8. TRACHEOSTOMY.

8.1. TRACHEOSTOMY. BLOOD ASPIRATION IN HAEMATEMESIS.

A patient was brought from the casualty in a Stretcher, when I was in the ward. He is brother of a medical student. He vomited blood when he was being shifted from Stretcher to bed and devolved respiratory distress. A mouth gag was introduced we have transferred to I.C.U. in trauma ward. Myself and PGs. Were transported the patient and I asked the duty doctor in I.C.U.to pass the endotracheal tube first for the patient and apply suction. But the anaesthetist could not pass the endotracheal tube due blood and suggested tracheotomy. I did tracheostomy. In the meantime resuscitation was being done. Through the tracheostomy suction was applied. But in spite of all our efforts, the patient died. When we returned from I.C.U. the patient's wife, who was pregnant at that time asked us how is he. We could not answer that and we said he is in I.C.U., let us wait.

8.2. TRACHEOSTOMY IN OPERATION THEATRE CORRIDOR.

I had two occasions where tracheostomy was done in operation theatre corridor. Both were head Injury cases. In one case Dr.Perumal Raj PG Student was washing for tracheostomy in the theatre and the patient developed respiratory arrest when the patient is being shifted from ward to operation theatre. I just opened the trachea with an 11 Blade knife and kept open the tracheostomy opening by passing an artery forceps and followed the patient to the theatre and asked the PG. to complete the tracheostomy. Another case, I asked the nurse to prepare the table for emergency tracheostomy. When I went inside the theatre and saw the nurse is making the table as for any mayor surgery. When I am discussing with the nurse the patient become Cyanosed and Dr Jayachandran PG student did tracheostomy in the corridor itself. Professor A.A.A. used to say in dare emergencies you can do tracheostomy even with unsterile pen Knife and keep open the trachea opening will a hair pin. This statement is only to stress the urgency when a patient is in respiratory distress. We did tracheostomy with operating instrument to save the life.

My Chief Dr S.Shanmugam used say that the indication for tracheostomy is when the surgeon thinks that tracheostomy may help the patient is itself the indication for Tracheostomy. The indications for tracheostomy were tabulated by Mac Watts in 1960.

In those days of 1970 -1980 emergency tracheostomy were being done in all the cases of acute respiratory distress by the general surgeons. After eighties the needs of tracheostomy became rare due to endotracheal tube and ventilator. Even if tracheostomy is needed for prolonged endotracheal tube it is being done by E N T Surgeon and the general surgeons are not doing tracheostomy nowadays.

9. TETANUS.

9.1. TETANUS PATIENT REQUESTED PERMISSION FOR MARRIAGE.

A 25 years male was admitted for Tetanus. He had treatment for 3 days. Patient's relatives wanted permission for the patient to go out in the morning to attend marriage and they said they will bring the patient in the evening. I told them the condition is not fit to leave the hospital. They said he has to be there because it is his marriage. I said change the marriage date for 2 or 3 months later and refused to give permission to leave the hospital. He went against medical advice, had the marriage, and returned late in the evening to the ward. The ward nurse told them he was discharged against medical advice in the day time itself and so she cannot permit him to stay in the ward. If you wanted admission, go to the casualty and get admission slip so that she can keep him in the ward and inform the duty assistant for treatment. They went to casualty and got admitted as admitting unit case. Next day the other unite assistant send the patient's case sheet stating that you have treated the case and so take over the case. I wrote in the case sheet, if the patient has our unit op ticket he can be transferred to our care otherwise treat as a new case, where was admitted yesterday night. As the patient had some improvement with 3 days of active treatment, they thought he will be improve after sometime and so they took him for his marriage and after the marriage functions were over, as the time passes, the effect of the drugs given to the patient before he leaves the hospital has gone and the symptoms recurred. So they brought the patient in the evening for the treatment.

9.2. LADY HOUSE SURGEON CLAIMED THE NEEM TREE.

When our unit lady house surgeon went to Tetanus ward, one patient had severe spasm due to tetanus and had respiratory distress. She asked for airway or at least the mouth gag just open the mouth and keeps it open for breathing through the mouth. The ward nurse told her that both are not available. Immediately she went out and claimed the nearby Neem tree and broke a reasonably large branch of the tree cut it to the size of mouth gag rolled it with gauze and put it in to the mouth of the patient and kept for some time, the respiratory distress reduced. In the meantime she asked the nurse to give muscle relaxant and sedation and saved the patient. When I went for night rounds she told me about what has happened in the Tetanus ward. I appreciated her timely action and her presence of mind. Next day I went to Dean's office with her and told the incidence and the Dean Dr.Parvathi Devi also appreciated her. I asked the nurse to get airway and mouth gag from the stores for the Tetanus ward.

9.3. NURSES WERE ON STRIKE FOR AN INCIDENT IN TETANUS WARD.

On those days Tetanus patients are treated on the floor only. In our admission day one case of Tetanus was admitted in tetanus ward. The duty house surgeon saw the case and wanted to start the treatment immediately. So he asked the nurse to bring drips set and 5% Dextrose saline. The nurse said they are not available in the ward. So the house surgeon brought the saline bottle and drip set from the main ward. In those days I.V Solutions were prepared in the hospital itself and supplied to the ward. The reusable I.V sets are sterilized in the hospital. They are supplied in limited number to each ward. After struggling for some time the I.V drip was started with the help of the patient's relatives and the house surgeon asked the nurse to bring plaster to fix the drip set and saline stand to hang the bottle. The nurse said both are not available. The house surgeon got angry, and slapped the face of the nurse in the ward in the presence of patients and attenders. He got the plaster from the main ward and made some arrangements to hang the saline bottle. The house surgeon has not told the incidence to the duty assistant. The nurse complained to the Nursing Association. Next day the secretary of the Nursing Association demanded apology from the House surgeon but he refused to get apology. When I came for night rounds the house surgeon was in the post operative ward. After completing the rounds the House surgeon said that he wanted to talk with me and said what has happened on the admission day and the demand from the secretary of nursing association for apology. Then I went to tetanus ward and saw the patient and discussed will the patient's relatives in tetanus ward and gathered the information about the incidence. Everybody said the nurse behaved very badly with that doctor. I informed my Chief Dr C. Kalidoss about it in the nigh itself. The matter has gone to DME. He came on the next day morning. He had discussion with the nursing association and then called for a meeting with Assistant surgeons in the auditorium. The DME in his introductory speech said what the nursing association has said. But it was entirely different from what has happened and what I heard from the patients and their attendees on the previous day.

DME repeatedly asked why, why and why such a thing has happened. Everybody kept silent. I said because the non availability of proper things in tetanus ward. The DME said you were not on the spot and saying the information gathered from third persons. I said Sir; you were also not in the spot and telling the one side version. I went to the tetanus ward and enquired with all the patients and attenders. Then the DME said you sit down. Other doctor sitting near to me made me to sit. Now the DME said I will see all necessary items are available in tetanus ward and the meeting was closed abruptly.

9.4. POST OPERATIVE TETANUS.

A patient from a remote village from nearby Madurai was operated for Piles in G.R.H. When I went for night rounds in 2nd Post operative day he removed the dressing and used dirty cloth to cover the wound. I scolded him for using dirty cloth for dressing. He said the dressing has fall down so I used it. I changed the dressing in the night. He was discharged on the 6th day as routine. After 3 weeks one person was waiting in the main ward at 8-30 AM. I could not recognize him. The ward nurse said he was the person who used his own cloth for dressing. When I saw his face I made the diagnosis of Tetanus. I told him that it is because you used your own cloth for dressing which was not sterilized. He has not bought the discharge summary record but I know that he is our patient and traced old record I gave another discharge summary and admitted him in Tetanus ward. He has completely recovered. This is because the house surgeon in change of tetanus ward looked after the patient well.

9.5. TETANUS PATIENT TREATED IN THE MAIN WARDS.

The management of Tetanus was changed from 1990 onwards the patients need not be isolated and he can be treated in a bed. But separate Syringes, dressings to be used. Of course nowadays the disposal syringes are being used and one time dressing packs are available. Many papers were published recording this. The incidence of tetanus was also reduced. I have admitted a case of tetanus in main ward. It was with minimal symptoms and I asked the nurse to provide a corner bed. The nurse opposed and gave a complaint to the nursing Superintendent. By this time I am the unit chief. The Dean called me and asked about it. I showed him 5 or 6 literatures and said tetanus patients need not be isolated and moreover it is only a mild case. If treated in tetanus ward the patient will die because of poor care of the patient. In the main ward the medical and nusing cares will be good and the patient can be discharged without any complications. The Dean said you may be right in treating in main ward but the convention is Tetanus patients should be isolated. Anyhow let the patient be in the main ward till discharge and hereafter do not admit Tetanus patient in main ward. Fortunately no Tetanus patient was admitted in my admission day afterwards. The overall incidence of tetanus is markedly reduced.

10. INTRACTABLE ASCITES DUE TO CIRRHOSIS LIVER.

10.1. VARIOUS TYPES OF OPERATIONS TRIED FOR PALLIATION.

If you want to be best you have to do things that other people are willing to do.

In those days the treatment for ascites was the use of diuretic and periodic aspiration of ascetic fluid. This results in hypo proteinemia and electrolytes imbalance. After going through the recent advances in the management of ascites, I did various methods like omentopexy, multiple scaring in the peritoneum for the omental adhesions. Peritoneo Sephenous shunt using Uppadyaya Shunt though it works well the early Stage, Shunt got blocked within one month. Thoracic duct internal jugular vein anatomises was tried. Later Levin shunt was used for Peritoneo venous drainage of the ascetic fluid in to the circulation. The question is how to get the best from everything. Initially the Shunt caused Rs 4500 and gradually increased to the level of Rs 25000. The hospital administration refused to buy such a costly shunt for palliative measures.

10.2. PERITONEO VENOUS SHUNT.

After doing three cases, it was presented in Clinical Society meeting. There were heated arguments about the quantity of urine output after surgery. I said in the post operative period the urine output was 4 to 4.5 litres within 24 hours. The audience did not accept this high volume of urine output and one person said the patient cannot live with such high urine output. I explained the reason for such a high amount of urine output, as the ascitic fluid being shunted to circulation, resulting in high volume of circulation and diuretic were given to reduce the circulative volume. I also said all 3 patients are alive after the Shunt and you can see them here. One patient treated by shunt has donated one ceiling fan to the ward and said it must be fixed over the bed when he was in the hospital.

10.3. POST DEVASCULARSATION ASCITES.

I did devascularisation of stomach and oesophagus for severe, repeated, haematemesis due to Portal hypertension as the result of Cirrhosis Liver. After 16 months he developed ascites and came to the ward where I was working during his previous surgery. The surgeon in the ward told him that Doctor was transferred and he examined the patient and told him nothing could be done now. The patient went home and attempted suicide. Fortunately he was saved by local people. He told the people he cannot live with such a distended abdomen. One person in the crowd, told him to see Dr.Sivalingam and the patient told them that he only operated me 16 months back and now he left the hospital. Another man told him the doctor is in ward 221. Now he came to ward 221 with distended abdomen and he showed the old records. He could not even walk due to ascites. I explained his nature of surgery and its risks, which I am going to do. He agreed for the shunt and said even if I die no matter, I cannot live with this distended abdomen. Peritoneo venous shunt was done using Levein shunt. He went home happily and came for review after I month and he was quite comfortable now to move around.

10.4. PULMONARY OEDEMA AFTER PERITONEOVENOUS SHUNT.

One patient died following Peritoneo venous shunt due to pulmonary oedema as the result of over loading of fluid in circulation. The house surgeon was newly posted and he was by the side of the patient till the death of the patient. He has not consulted the PG and not informed me also. When I came for the night rounds I saw the bed was empty. I asked the duty House surgeon what has happened. He said the patient suddenly developed respiratory distruss and died within 20 minutes and I was with the patient all the time. If he has consulted the P.G. or contacted me the patient would have been saved. If his House surgeon was not in the ward, the nurse would have contacted me by phone and I would have given some instructions. Whatever may be to me it was a preventable death.

10.5. PORTO SYSTEMIC DISCONNECTION.

I have operated 3 lady patients with Portal hypertension with haematemesis. I did Porto Systemic Disconnection (Grill operation) Ligating the blood vessels supplying the Proximal part of the stomach and distal part of the oesophagus. This will reduce of blood to the portal system, reduces the size of the oesophageal veins and the bleeding will Stop. Of those 3 patients, one patient had divorce and her husband married to another lady. One patient became pregnant after 2 years. When she came with pregnancy I told her, have delivery in a hospital and not in the home. She said I will inform you when I am going to get admitted in G.R.H or my husband will inform you. She also said that I must see her in the hospital before delivery and inform the doctor about the nature of surgery she had. I told her that I will come and see you but you must show all the previous records to the doctor in the labour ward. The patient had normal delivery. The 3rd patient came for review for 2 months only and last to follow-up.

11. HERNIA.

11.1. OBSTRUCTED INGUINAL HERNIA. NOT FIT FOR ANAESTHESIA.

The main ward House surgeon informed about the admission of obstructed inguinal hernia, and all the investigations were already done. On that day we had 4 emergencies and we were operating from 3 PM onwards to 3 AM. I went to the ward and saw the case. He needs immediate surgery. So I asked the nurse to send the case to operation theatre immediately. By this time the last case was over. I told the anaesthetist about this case and showed all the investigations. She is a senior person and she was also tired. She saw the case before I transfer the patient from Stretcher to operation table and wrote in the case sheet that the patient is unfit for anaesthesia. I agree all are tired and we are in the theatre from 3 PM onwards. Any how we have to do surgery. So I wrote in the case sheet that this patient needs immediate surgery and I will do under local and take all the responsibility if anything happen to the patient. You give supportive management for the patient in the form of sedation and oxygen supplementation. Now the anaesthetist told me I am very tired, you proceed with the surgery under local and ask your P.G. to give sedation and O2, you can call me at anytime. She might have told me this before writing in the case sheet and we would have done under Spinal. On those days I.V drip starting, pre medications and spinal anaesthesia are given by the operating team. The operation went on successfully and the post operative period was smooth and the patient was discharged.

I am not finding fault with the anaesthetist because she was also with us in the theatre all the time and giving anaesthesia and surgical team will change for the cases. The operation theatre work is a combined responsibly. But because the team is tired we cannot postpone emergency surgery and put the life of the patient under risk.

11.2. OBSTRUCTED INGUINAL HERNIA. DEMONDED SURGERY BY ME.

Govt. Rajaji Hospital X Ray department attender came to the operation theatre and told the operation theatre assistant that he wanted to me. I was just washing for a case in the theatre. Many of the hospital servants will see me for treatment in outpatient department. That day was not our admission day. I came out and saw him. He said he has severe abdominal pain and I must see him. I examined him in a Stretcher. He had obstructed inguinal hernia which needs immediate surgery. I told him about the need for immediate surgery and get admitted in admitting Unit. He said you must do the surgery. I told him that he must go to casualty and get admitted in the admitting unit of that day. Today is not our admission day. He said if you are not operating me, I will not go to other unite and I will die without operation. I told my chief Dr.Kalidoss and he said admit him in our unit and you operate after our theatre works are over.

He was admitted in our ward and surgery was done in the afternoon before my lunch. The patient was a very sincere worker in X-ray department so I helped him. Moreover he said he will die if I don't operate him which made me to operate him.

11.3. OBSTRUCTED INGUINAL HERNIA SURGERY AFTER 6 DAYS.

I saw a case of obstructed inguinal hernia in Dr. Fenn hospital in the night and told the patient that he needs emergency surgery. I told Dr. Fenn that next day morning I am going to Goa for my F.I.C.S. Convocation so my service may not be available for another 6 days. The patient was also not willing for surgery and he went against medical advice. After I returned from Goa Dr. C.Rajasekaran general Practitioner called me to see a case that is waiting for the past 2 days. I saw the patient and I could identify the patient and the patient also recognized me. These 2 days he was on nil oral and iv fluids, antibiotics, and sedation. The patient was hypertensive and was treated by Dr. Rajasekaran. After came out from Dr. Fenn hospital the patient was in his home in Lakshmi Puram 5th street for 3 days and then got admitted in Dr. Rajasekaran clinic. I examined the patient and now I suspected gangrene of the bowel. I discussed with Dr. Rajasekaran about the patient that I have seen him 6 days earlier before I went to Goa. I thought that he could have surgery at that time. Now I suspect gangrene, on the death may occur. But he needs surgery. We are here to do something to the patient with risk and we should not say nothing could be done. Both of us explained the need for surgery and all about the risks and even table death to the relatives of the patient. They agreed for surgery and the patient also agreed because of the suffering. They asked me which hospital I am going to operate. I said Vadamalayan hospital. The patient's wife requested me to operate in a hospital near our house so that anything happens we take home without any difficulty. Dr. Rajasekaran said we can operate in Dr. V.N.R. hospital which is in East Masi street. I told Dr. Rajasekaran to talk with DR. VNR if he permits I will talk with him. Dr. VNR agreed and then I discussed with him about the risks and even table death. He said so far there was no table death in our operation theatre and so you proceed with confidence. Anaesthetist said the patient is not fit for any type of anaesthesia, you do the surgery under local and I will support the patient by sedation and O2 supplementation. I took the challenge and operated under local and resected 4 inches of small bowel. To a surprise to everyone the patient did well in the post operative period. The following week was Diwali day; the patient's daughter brought a bucket full of Diwali sweets to me and said because of me they are celebrating Diwali.

11.4. POOR RISK CASE. WANTED SURGERY BEFORE KUMPABISHEGAM.

A 60 year old man from nearby Karaikudi came to me with Irreducible inguinal hernia. He was known diabetes, hypertension, and had one heart attack treated by Dr. V. Srinivasan Honorary physician Govt. Erskine hospital (now Rajaji hospital). I told the patient that it is an irreducible hernia, may go for obstruction at any time and because of medical conditions and previous heart attack you need 3 or 4 days to stay in the hospital for controlling the diabetes and hypertension. I will call your Doctor Dr. Srinivasan to see you. The patient said he is the Chairman of the committee of Kumpabishegam of the temple in his village which to be held in the next month. I told him that this irreducible hernia may go for obstruction at any time. In that case emergency surgery has to be done without controlling the diabetes and hypertension. Dr. Srinivasan also said the same thing. So the patient agreed for surgery. He said he will live after surgery and he will be in the temple for Kumpabishegam and so you do the surgery. He had surgery after controlling the diabetes and hypertension.

The patient went home without any complication. I asked him to consult Dr. Srinivasan for further management. He invited me for Kumpabishegam but I couldn't attend.

11.5. OBSTRUCTED HERNIA OPERATED ON THE DAY OF DAUGHTER'S BETROTHAL.

I saw a case of inguinal hernia in my clinic and advised surgery. He said people were coming to see his daughter for marriage on the next day and he is hopeful that Betrothal date will be fixed on that day itself. So I will come after Betrothal. I said this hernia may get obstruction at any time and in that case surgery has to be done as emergency. Delaying surgery is up to you and later you should not say that you only permitted to come after Betrothal. The Betrothal function went on with classical village convention in the night. He also took the meals and when he was talking with the people around him he had 3 or 4 bouts of sneezing and the hernia got Obstructed. He came to Vadamalayan hospital at about 1 AM. Since he has taken heavy metal at about 9 PM immediate surgery cannot be done under anaesthesia. The foot end of the bed was raised, sedation was given and ice packs were applied over the hernia. He was investigated and surgery was done at 6AM under spinal. Everything went on well. When he came for review I asked what the bride groom side peoples said about the incidence. He said some ladies said something about this and now no problem. The moral from this case is when you see a case of hernia, you strangly advice surgery. Usually the patients want to post pone for 6 months or one year saying that they have some important works to do. Then tell them that it is on their own risk they are postponing surgery and later they should not find fault with the surgeon. An emergency surgery is strain to the patient and the family members. They may say that if you have said strongly I would have agreed for surgery at that time itself.

11.6. A MILITARY EXSERVICE MAN WITH MULTI VALVULAR DISEASE.

A military Ex service man came to my Clinic with large inguinal hernia. He had multi valvular disease of the heart. He told me that he has seen so many surgeons including two ex military surgeons regarding this condition. They refused to do surgery because of the heart disease. One of his friends directed him to see me and gave my address. He said cannot sleep peacefully when I have pain in that area and he requested me to operate him. I told him that it is a high risk case. He said even if die on the table I am prepared so please do surgery. I told him that death may occur on the table and if your family members agree I take the risk and operate. His family members also agreed. Surgery was done with monitoring and he was kept in the ICU for proper postoperative care. Alternative sutures were removed on the 4th post operative day by me and I told him that I will remove the rest of the sutures on the 6th post operative day and discharge on the 7th day. But I was admitted in the same ICU on his 6th post operative day. I was told later that when he was discharged after suture removal, he saw you through the glass doors and said that you were saying that he may die on the table but now I am going home and he is in I.C.U. and he will also be alright. He came for review after 2 months. I asked him why he has not come earlier whether you thought that I would have died. He said I know that you were not died, if died it would have come in the paper and now I have come to see you back.

11.7. MY AMBITION IS TO GET BLACK BELT.

A Male person was referred to me for inguinal hernia surgery. As the patient enters into my clinic he said his ambition is to get the black belt in karethae. I said for that you have to visit other places and not to me. He said no sir I was told that I have hernia and must have surgery for that. Can I practice for black belt after surgery? I told him first let me examine you and then we can discuss. When I examined him in lying position, and in standing position, I was not able to find out the hernia. I asked him to go fast to Meenakshiamman temple, have the Darson of Vibuthy pillaiyar and bring some vibuthy for me. He came within Half an hour. I examined him both in standing and lying position. As such I was not able to find out the hernia. Any how you practice karethae, and now also I could not find out hernia. I told him come after one month. After one month he came, and even now I was not able to find out the hernia. I asked him to continue his practice and take part in the competition for Black belt. If you have any swelling in the groin immediately come to me. He came after 3 months and showed me the black belt. After 6 months he asked me whether he can marry, I examined this time also and then I said yes Proceed. He came to me after 2 years with a Male child with his wife just to say thanks to me. In this case if I operated on suspicions of hernia, he would not have continued the practice and his whole life would have been spoiled. Later he started Karethae School in Madurai.

11.8. UTERUS IN INGUINAL HERNIA IN A, 'MALE'.

A 20 years male was admitted for right side undescended testis with hernia. After investigations he was posted for surgery. PG student was doing the case. When the inguinal canal was opened the sac could not be separated and the PG was in a confused state. One PG (Dr. Thangamuthu) came to me and drew a diagram and asked me Sir is it uterus, tube and ovary. I asked him why you have such a fundamental question. He told me it is exactly the findings in that undescended testis with hernia case. I saw the field of surgery, what he said was correct. There was no testis.- instead the uterus, Tube and ovary were seen. I joined the team and excised the whole mass and herniorrhaphy was done. I opened the inguinal canal in the left side, where the testis was seen in the scrotum, was normal. In the excised specimen I marked the so called uterus and ovary separately and sent to histo pathological examination. The Biopsy report came as uterus and the other one as ovo testis (the histological appearance of both ovary and testis). We took the patient to Madurai Kamaraj University for genotype. They said the genotype of the patient is Male. As the patient has both testis and ovary it is the typical case of Intersex like Arthanareeswarar. Because of rarity this case was presented in clinical society meeting and also published in the journal and this was my first paper publication.

11.9. NO ATTENDANT—SURGERY WAS NOT DONE.

A case of inguinal hernia with diabetes and hypertension was admitted for surgery. After stabilizing both, surgery was planned. On the day of surgery when I entered the operation theatre, there was no attendant in the theatre veranda. I asked the nurse about this. She said the patient told that his son will come soon and so we brought the patient to the theatre. Now I asked the patient why his son has not come yet. The patient said my wife was not doing well for the last 3 or 4 days and now she may be in a serious condition. Anyhow he will come now. We were waiting for more than 30 minutes. His son had not come and so we have cancelled the surgery and told the patient that surgery will be done on the next day. The patient compelled me to operate. I told him if something happened to you what we will do, definitely I will do surgery tomorrow and asked the theatre assistant to transfer the case to the ward. When I was going to my scooter patient's son has come. I asked him why he was late. He said his mother was in serious condition due to diabetes and I was with her. I asked him then why he came now. He said I thought that the surgery for my father would have been completed so I came here to sit by the side for some time. I told him surgery was not done because no attendant for him in the hospital. I will do surgery tomorrow. Next day surgery went on well and the patient was discharged after 5 days. The patient came for review after 10 days. After examination of the patient and advice, I was waiting for the information about his wife and finally I asked him about his wife's condition. He said she is alright and she had such a situation twice previously. That is why I asked you to do surgery. But you did on the next day.

11.10. SAME OPERATION BUT DIFFERENT CHARGES.

Both husband and wife were teachers in Primary school, brought their only son for consultation. I examined him and said he has inguinal hernia and needs surgery. In those days (1980s) the teachers pay was low. They said they were not financially well, because he is the only child we wanted the surgery to be done in private hospital and we did not want to go to GRH. They asked me what will be the total expenditure. I said the rough estimation. They bargained in a sympathetic way. I said I can reduce my Bill but whatever the hospital charges you have to pay. They took A- Type room in the hospital though B type of rooms and common type were available at that time which were relatively low rates. On the same day I operated another patient of inguinal hernia, who was related to a nurse working in GRH. For both the cases the nurse gave my Bill. As promised to the teacher couples may Bill was lesser than the other patient who is related to the nurse. The teachers couples compared the bill and told the nurse ask the doctor why there is difference in the bill though the surgery was same. The nurse said the doctor is always considering all aspects before billing and your surgery may be different. There was some discussion regarding my Bill, finally Vadamalayan hospital nurse said why you bother about the other person's bill and your bill is less than the other patient. Finally they paid the bill and got discharged. When I came for the rounds in the next day morning the nurse told me about the incident. I told her that they begged to do surgery as minimal as possible and so I reduced the amount. But they have taken A type of room which is highest rated.

I will ask them when they come for review. After 10 days they came for review. I examined the patient and gave the advice. I asked the parents why you compared my Bill for identical surgery. I charged less for you because you begged to reduce the operation charge as minimum as possible so I reduced my charge and I did as I promised. By seeing the bill you would have been happy that I kept my promise. But you took the costly room and you were prepared to spend for your comfort. That is alright, why you instigate the other person to ask for reduction of my Bill. You have no right to talk like that to our nurse that I have charged more. In fact if you are a straight forward man you should have asked the nurse why your Bill is less. The nurse knew all about the reasons and she would have explained. Then they got apology for their behaviour. Billing by the doctor depends upon so many factors which you cannot question.

11.11. DIAPHRAGMATIC HERNIA.

A case of intestinal obstruction with classical findings was admitted through causalty. The patient was investigated and surgery time was fixed at 9 PM. Final year students came for the evening Clinic. This patient was shown to them and the clinical discussion was going on the patient started shouting with pain. I immediately cancelled the clinical demonstration and asked the nurse to shift the patient to the operation theatre. I told the anaesthetist (Dr. Santhinathan) that is a straight forward case of volvulus sigmoid and we will finish the surgery within half an hour. He said you surgeons say like that if the time is prolonged you say some excuses. Anyhow I give general anaesthesia. We started the case, as predicted by him it was not a case of volvulus sigmoid. It was a case of left side diaphragmatic hernia where the sigmoid colon had gone up to the thorax. The sigmoid was brought down to the abdomen; fortunately there was no gangrene of the bowel. The defect in the diaphragm was closed and the abdomen was closed. Sometimes it happens like this the: operative findings may be entirely different from our clinical diagnosis. I have published a paper on Laparotomy delight and disappointment in1976. At that time Ultra sonogram, CT and MRI services were not available in GRH and that was the situation in many centres in India. I saw CT in1981 when I was doing Common Wealth Medical Fellowship in England. Now these services are available in every centres.

12. INCISIONAL HERNIA.

12.1. CAME FOR SURGERY IN THE FIRST DAY OF CONSULTATION ITSELF.

A lady from Rajapalayam came to my Clinic for consultation for incisional hernia with previous medical records. She had 4 surgeries previously, LSCS, abdominal hysterectomy, and two incisional hernia repairs. After examination I told her that she needs mesh for her hernia repair. She said she is prepared for surgery. I told her discuss with your family members and get admitted in Vadamalayan hospital. She said family members have come and I will get admitted today itself and you do the surgery according to your convenient. I called her family members. Some 4 or 5 people came and said she was seen in some other hospital in Madurai and we have come to get admitted in that hospital. The patient said that I told my neighbour to look after my house as I am going to Madurai for surgery. The neighbour told her that you already had four surgeries; you better consult Dr. Sivalingam who is in East Veli street, Madurai. You see him if he agrees to do surgery then get operated by him, if he refuses to do surgery for you, don't have surgery in other hospital, you come back. It seems she knows me. So this patient has come to me. Really I was happy to hear that word and I appreciated that lady directed her with faith and confident upon me.

12.2. INCISIONAL HERNIA. PATIENT DEMANDED I MUST DO SURGERY.

In 18.2.1999 at about 6.30 AM I got information from my Brother about my mother's death. I told him I will be starting at 9AM after the driver comes. My wife Dr. Balasaraswati has gone to Vadamalayan hospital to see a delivery case at 5AM. When I was about to inform her mother's death, she rang up to me and called me for emergency LSCS for that case. I went and after finishing the surgery I told her the death of my mother and we have to start at 9 o'clock today. When I came back from the operation theatre a school teacher with severe abdominal pain, was waiting for me. She was known to me for some time. I examined her, she had obstructed incisional hernia. I told her that she needs immediate surgery. She agreed for the surgery and said you must do the surgery. I told her that I can't operate her now, and if you have come here for me I will ask some other doctor to operate. If you have come to Vadamalayan hospital, get admitted as hospital case and they will make arrangement for the operating team. She said she has come here only for me. Then I told her about my mother's death. She said you suggest the doctor for surgery, I will be admitted as your case. I talked with Dr. Mahadevan about the situation and i asked him to operate the case as early as possible. He operated the case and looked after the case till I returned from Mukkudal. As I told my brother that I will be starting from Madurai at 9AM. he waited till 1PM and rangup to Vadamalayan hospital to find out what time I have started. The receptionist replied that we left the hospital only at 9AM. They were waiting for our arrival for further arrangements for the funeral. There was no cell phone service at that time.

12.3. SURGERY PREFIXED BECAUSE OF OBSTRUCTION.

A patient from Kumbam Cudalore was admitted for incisional hernia. Surgery was fixed at 3.30 pm as elective surgery. On the Previous night the patient had obstruction and the duty doctor informed me informed me at 1.30 am. I asked him to record Pulse BP and abdominal girth measurement and also advised to give antispasmodic drug and sedation. He again called me and said pain still continued and the abdominal girth increased for 5 cm. Since the patient was prepared for surgery and in starvation I told him fix for surgery at 6AM and tell the patient and the relatives. After checking the theatre register he said at 6 am another surgeon had fixed for surgery. Then I told him I will start the case at 4.30 am and tell the theatre nurse and fix up the anaesthetist. My wife Balasaraswathi assisted, I finished the operation and left the hospital before 6 AM (before the other surgeon comes).

12.4. OBSTRUCTION ON THE NEXT DAY OF SON'S MARRAIGE.

Mr. Dhanabal met with accident and liver injury for which I operated him in 1992. He devolved incisional hernia. Surgery for incisional hernia was fixed in 1999 after pongal. But endotracheal tube could not be passed due to some reason and the patient developed pulmonary oedema. So surgery was not done. Later his son's marriage was fixed I couldn't attend the marriage. Three days after the marriage his wife was standing in the veranda in Vadamalayan hospital. I asked her about the marriage and asked her to bring the couple to my house one day and asked how is Dhanabal. She said he is admitted here and we are waiting for you. I asked the nurse what time he was admitted. The nurse said the patient was admitted at 8 am, because you will be coming at 8.30 am I have not informed you. The duty doctor has seen the case and ordered for the investigations and started IV fluid. I saw the patient, the incisional hernia got obstructed. I asked him how long he had pain. He said in the next day of marriage at the time of maruveedu I had some pain but somehow I was managing, once the function was over I came here to day morning. I asked the nurse to collect the blood reports and all reports were normal. The surgery was fixed at 3.30 pm in the same day. I informed the anaesthetist about the difficulty in intubation on the previous occasion. Luckily this time endotracheal tube could be passed without any difficulty. The incisional hernia repair was done with mesh. The post operative period was uneventful. In the meantime the recently married couple came to the hospital and they thanked me for the surgery

12.5. INCISIONAL HERNIA, POST OPERATIVE HEMIPLEGIA.

GRH Pharmacist daughter had incisional hernia which was operated by me in Vadamalayan hospital. The patient's mother is a nurse in GRH. She worked in our ward and in the operation theatre also. On the 5th post operative day the patient developed some weakness in the left upper Limb at about 6 am. The parents came at about 8 am and the duty nurse informed me. I asked her to contact Dr.Neethiarasu neuro physician and asked him to see the case before my morning rounds. When I went to the hospital Dr. Neethiarasu has seen the case. He said since the hemiplegia was diagnosed very early, the possibility of full recovery will be good. Since the hemiplegia occurred on the 5th post operative day I asked him to treat the patient as his case, I will remove the sutures on the 8th day. The patient needs no special treatment for the hernia repair. This I told him because he can have free hands to treat the patient. The patient started recovery from the 4th day of attack and almost recovered from hemiplegia.

12.6. RECURRENT INCISIONAL HERNIA. TREATED CONSERVATIVES.

A doctor was admitted in my unit for intestinal obstruction due to adhesions. He was operated for acute appendicitis and later for adhesive intestinal obstruction twice previously. I examined him and formed the base line for follow up examination. I told the doctor that he has intestinal obstruction due to adhesions and an incisional hernia in the lower part of the scar and there is no evidence of vascular impediments (gangrene) so we can wait for some time. But the doctor wanted surgery. I told him if I operate now there is no grandee that adhesive obstruction will not occur. I asked the duty doctor to measure the abdominal girth every hour if there is increase in girth more than one centimetre, to inform me. Enema was given the result was fair. Conservative treatment was continued. Next day he was transferred to C class ward in the X-ray block. In the evening the in charge nurse rang up to me and said the doctor is talking to his son about the assets and commitment and told him that he will not live. I went to the hospital immediately and saw him. He is improving well and do not know why he said to his son like that. I had bad experiences, when a patient says he will die, he or she dies in that admission. But I don't want that sentiment in this case because he is improving well. I told him if you want surgery I can do it now it but there is no indication for surgery. I will see you in the night rounds and decide, and I advised one more dose of antispasmodic drug. When I came in the night rounds he was comfortable and said he passed motion with flatus. He was discharged without surgery and told him you can get admitted at any time, on any day in our unit. He was later promoted as professor of medicine in Madurai Medical College. He retired from service on superannuation.

13. BREAST.

13.1. CANCER BREAST. JEGADEESWARI.

Mrs. Jegadeeswari married 8 years back, become pregnant for the first time. When she was 8 months pregnant she noticed a mass in the left breast. She consulted a surgeon. He did FNAC and advised immediate surgery with termination of pregnancy. Somebody directed her to see me. She came with all investigations. I told her we can wait for 2 to 3 weeks till the baby gains a reasonable weight. we do surgery for both with the help of my wife Dr. Balasaraswathi. They asked me whether the tumour will spread if we wait for 2 to 3 weeks. I told them that this particular baby is a precious baby after 8 years of marriage. If we do surgery for the breast alone something may happen to the baby. Moreover the course of cancer is unpredictable. Post operatively she may need Radiation therapy and chemotherapy. I told her get admitted in Vadamalayan hospital after 2 weeks. We check the baby weight by Sonar study and when the baby gains an acceptable weight we can operate. They said we will discuss with other members of the family and come after 2 weeks. She was admitted after 2 weeks. Dr. Balasaraswathi followed the case for the baby weight and surgery date was fixed when the baby weight was in reasonable one in consultation with the patient and family members. My wife did Caesareans section and bilateral oophorectomy and then I did total mastectomy and axillary clearance. After 3 months when the baby has grown to some level, I thought she needs irradiation so she was referred to CMC Vellore. They were also of my opinion and she had irradiation and chemotherapy. After 5 years a nodule was noticed on the right breast by the patient and she came to me. I did core Biopsy and the report was malignancy. I told them about the need for surgery for that and the same line of treatment for this side also. They agreed for the surgery. When I am just entering the operation theatre, this child now 5 years talked with me, said you must save my mother. I said you gave been saved by me and so you do not worry. The patient was treated successfully with follow up chemo radiation. When the child attained menarche we attended the function.

Later her marriage was conducted in my presence at Madurai. When she became pregnant the delivery was conducted by my wife in Vadamalayan hospital. After 2 years she had 2nd pregnancy and the delivery was conducted by my wife. Now she was advised family planning surgery and it was done. In this case if surgery for the cancer Breast was done at 8 months of pregnancy prematurely they would not have a family varisu and now the family tree is maintained. Sometimes we have to undertake a compromised way in some particular situations.

13.2. RECURRENT FIBROADENOMA OF BREAST.

A teacher from near by Virudunagar (mrs.Padmalakshmi) came to me for a swelling in the left Breast. She was married 5 years back and no child. Clinically it was fibro adenoma. She was investigated and I thought I can do excision Biopsy under local. But the local infiltration of lignocaine had no effect on her. So the excision Biopsy was done under general anaesthesia. The Biopsy report confirmed fibro adenoma and no evidence of malignancy. She came after one year with recurrence on the same side. This time also there was no lignocaine effect. So she was operated under general anaesthesia. She was operated 5 times under general anaesthesia. I told her if you come again I have to remove the whole Breast. She came for the 6th time with recurrence. I did total mastectomy with preserve of the nipple and areola (sub areola resection) on 10.10.2006.

13.3. FIBROADENOMA OF BOTH BREASTS.

An unmarried girl was brought by her brother who was an assistant professor in a college for swelling in both Breasts. There was single swelling in both sides and clinically both swellings were fibro adenoma. I discussed with her Brother that it is not cancer but it may reoccur. When it recurs at that time don't get frighten as cancer. He agreed for surgery and I did excision of the fibro adenoma both sides under general anaesthesia. The Biopsy report Confirmed fibro adenoma. She came back after 2 years with swelling of same size in both sides like the previous time. She was operated and the Biopsy report confirmed fibro adenoma. Later her brother asked whether she can marry. I said yes, some time marriage and child birth may prevent recurrence. She got married and the delivery was conducted by my wife Dr.Balasaraswathi. After one year of child birth she came to my Clinic with her child and said she is working in the court as typist. I was happy to see the child and there was no recurrence of fibro adenoma.

14. THYROID SURGERY.

14.1. BLEEDING FROM THE WOUND.

A case of solitary nodule of thyroid was operated by the assistant. I was in the operation theatre till the hemi thyroidectomy steps were over. The operated wound has to be closed. I told the anaesthetist that I am going for a meeting in the hospital auditorium. When the anaesthetist about to remove the endotracheal tube, She noticed excessive bleeding from the drainage site. She asked the assistant to open up the wound and look for the site of bleeding. When the assistants were hesitating, she told them I will not remove the endotracheal tube unless you reopen the wound and she sent the theatre assistant to auditorium to inform me about the case. I used to sit in a particular place in the auditorium. The theatre assistant told me that the anaesthetist wanted me to come to the theatre. I reopen the wound and found the bleeding from the superior pedicle. I asked the assistant to ligate the superior pedicle again and close the wound. I thanked the anaesthetist Dr.Prema, a senior person in the department for informing me.

14.2. CANCER THYROID WITH LUNG SECONDARIES.

A well-known person in Madurai had thyroid swelling and advised surgery by many surgeons including myself. But he refused. His wife is also a leading gynaecologist, come to my clinic with X-ray chest of her husband with multiple lung secondaries. She asked me to talk with her husband. Their son and daughter in law are also doctors. I discussed with the patient, and family members, whatever may be the situation regarding the spread of the disease, he needs total thyroidectomy for further treatment. It has been reported that occasionally the lung secondaries may subside after total thyroidectomy. They agreed for surgery. In December 1988 surgery was done by me in their hospital. Dr. GnanaRaj M.D. and Dr. Shahul Hameed E.N.T Surgeon are also in the operation theatre. The post operative period was uneventful. After 1 year secondaries occurred in left Femur this was treated by Dr.Devadoss, the orthopaedic Surgeon, by excision of the secondary and used bone cements to fill up the gap. Later he developed spinal secondary and we could not save him.

15. COMPLICATIONS OF SPINAL ANAESTHESIA.

15.1. SPINAL SHOCK.

In Virudunagar Headquarter Hospital an emergency L.S.C.S. was started at 8.30 AM assuming that the case will be over before I come to the theatre, from outpatient clinic. It was delayed in starting the case due some problem. When I went to the theatre, the case was just started and skin incision was made and they were proceeding with the surgery. I changed the theatre dress and enter in to theatre. I noted that the patient is in Spinal shock and the anaesthetist was doing something to revive the patient. I asked him to pass the endotracheal tube and support the respiration. Also I asked the Surgeon to take out the baby as early as possible because she has already opened the abdomen. The baby was cyanosed and not crying. The paediatrician Dr.DuraiRaj came from outpatient and he passed tracheal tube and took other measures to revive the baby but the child could not be revived. By the time the surgery was over and abdominal wound was closed. The patient spontaneous respiration was not adequate. The D.M.O was informed and decided to refer to Govt Rajaji Hospital, Madurai. The patient was sent by ambulance with endotracheal tube and the anaesthetist accompanied the patient in the ambulance. I informed the chief anaesthetist about the case by phone and told him that the ambulance will come to G.R.H within 45 minutes. As the ambulance was nearing Thirumangalam, the respiration become adequate, but the endotracheal tube was not removed. The I.C.U. anaesthetist in Madurai examined the case and removed the endotracheal tube. The patient was kept in I.C.U. one day and transferred to gynec post operative ward and discharged after suture removal. The patient's husband and other relatives thanked us for the timely action to save the mother.

15.2. EPIDURAL ANAESTHESIA TURNED OUT TO BE TOTAL SPINAL.

A case of cancer penis posted for total amputation of penis. Epidural anaesthesia was given by Dr.R.Balachandran (R.B.C). When the patient turned to supine position, he noticed that total spinal anaesthesia had developed. Dr. R.B.C. in his own way of calmness passed the endotracheal tube and maintained the respiration. This case was supposed to be done by a PG and somebody else to assist him. I asked Dr.RBC whether a P.G. can do the surgery. He said anybody can do the surgery but you must assist them. So the PG (Jaya Singh Varghes) did the case and I assisted him. The surgery went on well and the patient started recovery from total spinal.

16. URGENT CALL FOR BLEEDING.

16.1. GRANULOMATOUS EPULIS.

A case of granulomatous epulis was posted for excision in E.N.T operation theatre by the dental surgeon. When he was doing excision there was severe bleeding. E.N.T Post graduate Student told me that I must come to E.N.T operation theatre immediately. At that time I was in the accident ward duty. I told the nurse and my P.G. that I am going to E.N.T. theatre for urgent call. I just opened the theatre door, the anaesthetist Dr.Padmalakshmi said change the operation theatre dress. I changing the dress and went in to the theatre, again Dr.Padmalakshmi asked me to scrub for the surgery and join the operating team. While I am scrubbing she told me it is a case of epulis had severe bleeding during surgery and so I called you. The operating area was packed well to control the bleeding till I joined the team. I slowly removed the pack. There was a gush of arterial bleeding and the source of bleeding could not be made out. So the external carotid artery was ligated in the neck and the bleeding was reduced and the dental surgeon had completed the surgery. Now I asked the dental surgeon how you called me. The anaesthetist said, Sir I know that you are in the accident ward and your service will be available all the time in accident ward during your duty time. So I only sent the E.N.T. P.G. to accident ward and bring you here. I considered it as a compliment for my work. Then I asked as per admission date which surgical unit the patient belongs. They said first surgical unit. I told him refer this case to first surgical unit for further management.

I will be in the ward on regular days up to 2 p.m. and then only I will leave the ward after telling the nurse and nursing assistance. So when a surgeon is required in the operation theatre, particularly in labour ward, they phone up to ward 218 for help.

16.2. URGENT CALL FOR CUTDOWN.

One of our admission days, the house surgeons and non service P.G. were on strike. The gynaec theatre assistant came to the O P and said Dr. Sivakamasundari wanted you to come to gyneac operation theatre immediately. I went there and asked what the problem was. Dr. Sivakamasundari was doing the surgery. She said change the theatre dress and come inside and do a cut down for this case as we have failed. I asked why you have started the emergency case without a drip or cut down. She said she tried in both legs so I called you. I used to do cut down in the upper limb only; I did cut down in the upper limb and established the IV line for IV fluid infusion and medications. It is said that it is a surgical sin to start IV line in the lower limb and so I avoid starting IV line in the lower limbs and do it in upper Limbs.

16.3. PORTAL HYPERTENSION STENSTAKAN TUBE PASSED.

A patient was admitted for severe haematemesis in the main ward. Dr. Kandasamy was on duty in main ward and I was in accident ward duty. Dr.Kandasany called me to see a case. It was a case of Portal Hypertension with haematemesis due to rupture of the Oesophageal verisis.

I passed the Stenstaken tube for compression of oesophageal verisis and aspiration of blood from the stomach. Stomach wash was given with normal saline till the return is clear, to find out any fresh bleeding after passing the tube. The tube was kept in position for 48 hours and gradually deflated and finally removed after 4 days after establishing there is no fresh bleeding. Somehow the bleeding had stopped and the patient was referred to medical side for further treatment. Later, after one year or so I went to Ibrahim stores near Meenakshi temple. This patient identified me and told that he was treated by me in GRH for vomiting blood. This patient developed pressure necrosis of the ala of the nose by Stenstaken tube fixed by the tape, by which I could remember that patient.

16.4. LUMBAR SYMPATHETCTOMY.

A case of T.A. O. was posted for Left Lumbar Sympathectomy. I was doing the case in the main table and my chief was doing some other minor case under local on the side table. While I am doing that left lumbar sympathectomy there was a gush of arterial blood. I thought I have injured abdominal aorta. I packed the area with abdominal pads and told my chief that I suspect I have injured abdominal aorta and packed that area, I need your help. He asked the other assistant to complete his case and scrubbed again and came. He slowly removed the pack one by one and when the last pack was removed, the bleeding was found from the pulsating lumbar branch of abdominal aorta which was ligated. Now my Chief said Sivalingam I appreciate your calmness and asked for the help instead of trying to catch the bleeder and ultimately injuring the aorta. This is how you must manage when there is unexpected arterial bleeding pack the area wait for some time and remove the pack slowly.

17. URINARY BLADDER AND URETHRA.

17.1. RETENTION OF URINE. S.P.C. PLANED PATIENT PASSED URINE.

When I was doing my senior P.G in 1969 one case of retention of urine was admitted. The bladder was distended up to the umbilicus and catheter could not be passed. The patient was prepared for Supra Pubic Cystostomy and transferred to operation table. Before injecting local anaesthesia in the abdomen, the patient said he has urgency to pass urine, we told him it will be possible to pass urine now we will let out the urine by operation. The patient ran away from the operation theatre, and passed urine near the operation theatre lift and he was quite comfortable after passing the urine and there was no bladder distension.

17.2. INTRA PERITONEAL RUPTURES OF BLADDER.

A patient was referred from Melur Hospital as retention of urine. The patient was in drunken status. On examination there was no bladder distension. When we asked the patient when he passed urine, he could not answer for that. There was tenderness in the supra public region. Catheterization was done only a few CC of blood stained urine was drained. X ray abdomen showed gas under the diaphragm. Emergency I.V. P was done. The Kidney excretion was normal in both sides and there is no evidence of Renal or ureter injury. As the patient had tenderness in the super pubic region and gas under the diaphragm, bowel Injury was suspected and the case was operated. The peritoneal cavity was found contaminated with blood stained fluid and Foley's catheter was seen in the peritoneal cavity coming from the doom of the bladder. So it is a case of rupture of the bladder due to fall with distended bladder. There was no other injury to the abdominal viscera. The bladder defect was closed and the Foley's catheter was connected to urobag. Now we were discussing how the gas under the diaphragm was seen in X ray. I asked the nurse when you have sent the patient for X-ray. She said immediately after you passed the catheter. When we saw the X -ray K.U.B area and the IVP the tip of the catheter was seen outside the bladder contour.

This incident remains the phrase that our eyes do not see what our mind does not know. Next day I showed the X Ray K.U.B and I.V.P. to the Radiologist he immediately said bladder rupture with Foley's catheter tip in the peritoneal cavity. The patient died on the 7th post operative day due to Pulmonary Embolism. We had another case of intra peritoneal rupture of the bladder in blunt injury abdomen, when I was in accident ward duty and he was successfully treated.

17.3. STRICTURE URETHRA WITH EXTRAVISATION OF URINE.

When we where in emergency operation theatre, the ward boy came to the operation theatre with case sheet and said one case of retention of urine is admitted. I sent a lady house surgeon to see the case and pass a catheter. After sometime she came back to the theatre and said his bladder was distended, and catheter could not be passed because he has a fungating lesion in the penis. As it is very rare for carcinoma penis involving the urethra, I changed my operation theatre dress, went to the ward and saw the case. It was a case of extravasations of urine due to stricture urethra. Multiple skin incisions were made and urethral dilatation was done and the catheter was kept in position for a week.

17.4. STRICTURE URETHRA - REPEATED URETHRAL DILATATION.

I still remember the patients Packrisamy and Gandhi. Both of them had urethral stricture and periodic urethral dilatation was done up to1981 after that I could not follow them as I left to U.K. for Common Wealth Medical Fellowship. They used to come on the previous day, had investigations and anaesthetic assessment and urethral dilation under short general anaesthesia on the next day as first case and discharged in the evening.

17.5. PRE-SACRAL DERMOID WITH URINARY RETENTION.

A 20 years male patient was admitted for difficulty in passing urine and feeling of heaviness in the perineum. Rectal examination showed a soft swelling between the Sacrum and Rectum. IVP was normal and the

Radiologist advised cystogram and it was fixed on the previous day of surgery. The house surgeon took the case for cystogram and he tried to pass the catheter in the X ray department but he could not pass in catheter. He called me. Catheter could not be passed by me also; the cystogram could not be done. The patient complained of not passed urine in the night. The duty doctor gave injection Lasix at about I AM for not passing urine. The patient developed distension of bladder extending up to the umbilicus. Duty doctor called me by phone at 2:30 AM. I told him to sedate the patient and tell him I will be seeing him at 8 AM. The patient was posted for surgery at 10 AM and blood was allotted for surgery, I do not want to do S.PC. Before going to the operation theatre I asked the patient whether he can wait up to 10' Clock for the chief to come. He said, he cannot wait so I informed my Chief Dr.C.Kalidoss and he said you start the case, I will be coming within 30 minutes. Under anaesthesia the catheter could be passed and the abdomen was opened. By that time Dr.C.K came and joined the team. The pre sacral dermoid was removed. On the 6th postoperative day the catheter was removed and the patient passed urine without any difficulty.

18. TUMOUR TESTIS.

18.1. TUMOUR TESTIS PRESENTED AS SECONDARY HYDROCELE.

A teaching staff member in Pharmacology department, madurai Medical College came to our ward for swelling in the Right Scrotum of I month duration. I examined him, it was a small secondary hydrocele with slightly enlarged testis and the testicular sensation was absent on the right testis. The epididymis was normal. Left side testis was normal. I suspected tumour testis. X ray chest and blood tests were done for anaesthetic assessment. I asked him to get admitted on the next day for surgery. I informed about the case to my chief Dr.C.K. The patient said it is harvest season in the paddy field and so I will come after the harvest. I just looked at him and I did not know what my facial expression was, he immediately agreed to come for admission. The case was operated by Dr.C.K. after the hydrocele fluid was let out the testis was examined. Externally it looks normal. The testis was split open along the outer border. A nodule was felt all the level of mediastinum of testis. So high architectomy was done and the specimen sent for Histopathological examination. The report came as seminoma. We referred him to Madras medical college Hospital for further evaluation and management. They gave irradiation for the Para aortic nodes. The patient lived for more than 15 years and he retired from service on superannuation.

18.2. TUMOUR TESTIS PRESENTED AS EPIDYDIMOARCHITIS.

MR. Muthuramalingam, Law college student and brother of Public relation officer, came to O.P for scrotal swelling on the left side of one month duration. On examination the left testis and epididymis were found thickened and tender, there was secondary hydrocele. No lymph node enlargement in the body. I suspected tuberculous epidydimo architis and admitted him for investigations and surgery. Under spinal, incision was made in the left side of the scrotum. When the Tunica vaginalis was incised multiple trabeculations were seen between tunica and the testis.

The tunica was excised and sent for Histopathological examination. I asked him to come after one week for suture removal and biopsy report. He came after one week sutures were removed. The biopsy report has not come at that time and so I asked him to come after 2 days.

After he left the ward, the biopsy report came and the report was Secondary deposits from tumour testis. I asked one of the senior house surgeons to go to law college hostel, find out his room number and if he is there bring him here. If he is not available in the room, tell his room mate that Dr.Sivalingam wanted to see him today. He came to the hospital at about 1.30 P.M. I explained the biopsy report and told him he needs another surgery and asked him to tell his brother and come for admission. He was admitted on the next day and high archidectomy was done on the following operation day. He had deep X-ray therapy for Para aortic region. He used to see me every month. In one visit he said he has breathlessness when he walks for some distance. I took X-ray chest. There was bilateral plural effusion. He was admitted on that day itself and plural aspiration was done on both sides. Check X Ray after aspiration showed multiple secondary in both sides. He died within a week.

19. OBSTETRIC AND GYNACE CASES.

19.1. ECTOPIC PREGNANCY.

When I was doing House surgeon in1965 I was in the outpatient clinic in maternity posting. I saw a case of ectopic pregnancy and admitted her in labour ward. The labour ward duty assistant said it is not ectopic and transferred the patient to the antenatal ward. Prof. K. BaskaraRao (K.B.R) saw the case in the night rounds and said it is ectopic pregnancy, transfer the case to labour ward and this case must be taken up for surgery immediately. The labour ward assistant now was different person, operated the case and it was ectopic and my diagnosis was correct. This was possible because I have worked is maternity department for 4 months when I failed in S.P.M. in final year examination. But the labour ward assistant said how a House surgeon can diagnose ectopic in outpatient clinic and because of that complex she has not examined the case properly and transferred the patient to the ward. The patient died on the 3rd post operative day. If she was operated immediately after admission, the patient could have been saved. No matter how great your words may be you will be judged by you action. Sometimes echo dominates at the expense of life in medical profession.

19.2. QUADRUPLETS DELIVERED BY LSCS.

A couple came to my wife for sterility. They were investigated and treated. The husband was assistant Professor in Agriculture College in Madurai. After some time she became pregnant. She had multiple pregnancies and was confirmed by abdominal scan, there were four foetuses. She was admitted in Vadamalayan hospital earlier than the expected date of delivery. It was decided to do LSCS once the membrane ruptured., One night the membrane ruptured the Anaesthetist and the Paediatrician were informed and all arrangements were made to receive the four Babies and for the resuscitation. Her husband has gone to Chennai for some meeting. I informed him about the surgery by phone. He said proceed with surgery I will come is the morning. Dr.Rathinasamy was the anaesthetist and I assisted the surgery. The babies were taken out from the uterus, 3 male and one female baby. The father of the new babies came in the morning. One baby named Nelson Mandela died after 3 days. The husband requested us not to report this in the media and not to give any interview. We said definitely we will not give any interview to the press, but if the matter comes out from hospital servants or relations of some other patients in Vadamalayan hospital, we are not responsible. They brought those 3 Children to my clinic after 2 years, they were very active and were playing in my clinic and I was very happy to see them.

19.3. OVARIAN CYST MISS INTERPRETED BY THE SONOLOGIST.

One doctor's Brother's wife was sent for abdominal scan and the doctor came to me with report and its pictures, the patient has not come. The report was ascites due to malignancy of the liver nothing could be done. It is wrong on the part of the sonologist to say about the treatment. They can say their findings and their opinion. I asked the doctor can you bring the patient. He said she is in my house only but I have not examined her. I asked the doctor to bring her to Vadamalayan hospital at 8-30 AM on the next day for examination. Next day I examined the patient and I had my doubt whether it is ascites at all. I thought it is a huge ovarian cyst on the right side. So the patient was send to gynaecologist, my wife, for pelvic examination. She is also of opinion that it is ovarian cyst but left side. I sent in patient to another scan centre for abdominal and pelvic scan. C.T or M.R.I was not available in Madurai at that time. I told the doctor if it is not ovarian tumour and only fluid in the peritoneal cavity, whatever may be the cause, abdominal tapping can be done so that the patient can sit down, walk to the toilet. The repeat scan report was ovarian cyst left side. After all the investigations we advised surgery for the patient. The surgery was done by my wife and I assisted her. She made a large left paramedian incision and with some difficulty the ovarian cyst was delivered out of the abdomen. The pedicle was long and so only three clamps were used and the left ovarian cyst was removed. Technically it was very simple. Examinations of other vicesera were normal the patient was discharged after 10 days. She was advised to wear abdominal belt. In this case the first sonologist was over confident about his Scan Interpretation. One can be confident in his findings, but should not be over confident.

19.4. STEIN LEVENTHAL'S SYNDROME.

Mrs. Papa from nearby Srivalliputhur was referred from gynaec department as Stein Leventhal's syndrome. The patient was married 15 years back and had no child. After all available investigations in 1973, the case was posted for Bilateral Subtotal Adrenalectomy. On laparotomy the uterus was found bulky and so it was decided to do subtotal hysterectomy also. After the uterine vessels were divided the uterus was incised the amniotic fluid came out. My chief asked the PG to call the gynaecologist to come to the theatre immediately. The gynaecologist came and my chief said you had missed the pregnancy and referred for adrenelectomy to us. The gynaecologist expressed the mistake. Bilateral Subtotal Adrenalectomy was done. The patient was discharged after suture removal. She came for 2 or 3 reviews and after that I have not seen her. In 1992 when I am retuning from my main ward rounds she was standing near surgery department office. I recognized her and asked her are you Papa? She was very happy that I have mentioned her name after so many years. I asked her why she has not come for follow up. She said she came twice and other doctors said you have gone to Foreign country (U. K) and another time when I came they said you have been transferred (Virudunagar). Today I asked the person in this office. He said he is here only, when he is coming from ward 221 you just say vanakkam. He will not talk to anybody when he is going to the ward. I saw you going to the ward and just kept quite as per his advice. After asking about her health, I asked what for she has come now. She said she developed diabetes and wanted to have treatment for that. I gave a reference letter to Dr.Kannan- endocrinologist and asked her to meet him in the outpatient clinic between10 - 1 2 Noon. Later Dr.Kannan told me that she was admitted for initial evaluation of diabetes and discharged her after establishing the dosage. I was very happy to see a case operated in 1973 and helped her in 1992 for the management of diabetes.

20. ACUTE APPENDICITIS.

20.1. FIRST CASE IN 1971 NEW YEAR DAY.

I was on duty in casuality on 31.12.1970 night. A boy by name Sikkander Basha, of about 15 years was brought to the casuality for acute abdominal pain. I asked the nursing assistant to take the boy to the bed. When I was about to raise from the chair to see the patient, the new year Bell rang from American college and other nearby churches and I told the nurse that this is the first case I am going to see in 1971. I examined the patient and it was a classical case of acute appendicitis. I admitted him and contacted the D.A.S (Dr. Gopalakrishnan) and told him I am admitting a case as New Year gift to you and tell me the findings after surgery. The D.A.S contacted me at 5 AM and said it was a case of acute appendicitis and it was about to bust out and carefully we did appendicectomy.

20.2. URETERIC COLIC PRESENTED AS ACUTE APPENDICITIS.

On our admission day the D.A.S. called me for a second opinion. I went to the hospital and saw the case. I am of opinion that it is a case of ureteric colic probably due to ureteric stone in the right ureter. So I told them let us wait till tomorrow morning, now you treat conservatively, give him antibiotics, antispasmodic and I.V. fluids. When I came for ward rounds, the patient showed me a small stone which he passed along the urine and he was more comfortable after passing the stone. It is a good thing that the D.A.S. wanted to have a second opinion as the patient was referred as acute appendicitis. On so many occasions I got second opinion from my chief.

20.3. ACUTE AMOEBIC COLITIS WAS MISTAKEN FOR ACUTE APPENDICITIS.

A male patient was admitted in our ward as acute appendicitis from casuality. I examined the patient all the symptoms and signs were of acute appendicitis. The only point was he had vomited more than 7-8 times which will not occur in acute appendicitis. Because the vomiting in acute appendicitis is a reflex phenomenon in which the vomiting may be 2-3 times only. I told the post graduate students that vomiting 7 to 8 times is only point against appendicitis but other clinical findings are classical for appendicitis. So let us take this case for surgery. Dr. Prema was the duty anaesthetist. She asked me who is going to do this case. I said it is a straight forward case so PG is doing it. She said who were maybe I will give general anaesthesia. Grid ion incision was made and at one stage they cannot find out the appendix and they called me. I said extend the incision above even then appendix could not be reached. The ileum is found inflamed and oedematous. The mesentery is also thickened and oedematous. Now I joined the team and made a low Para median incision. Again we were not able to find the appendix because of oedematous ileum and adhesions with inflammatory exudates. Even the touch of the ileum may lead perforation. So I accepted my defeat and closed the abdomen with corrugators rubber drain without doing appendectomy. (On those days we use corrugated rubber drain only). Next day two or more assistance in surgical side asked me about this case and asked is it such a difficulty to trace out the appendix? On the 3nd day when the dressing was changed I found exuberant granulation tissue at the site of drainage. I asked the P. G. to take a smear from the granulation tissue and look for amoeba. Within a few minutes the P.G. said there are plenty of amoebas, which I also confirmed. So anti amoebic treatment was given and the patient became alright. Perhaps our team persons are the only people who saw the pathological appearance of amoebic inflammation in ileum and caecum in a live person and amoebic granuloma of abdominal wall.

In this case I have accepted my inability to find the appendix as I felt that a life problem is better than the death certainty. If I made an attempt to find out the appendix I would have perforated the ileum and the peritoneal cavity would have been contaminated and I would have lost the patient.

By closing the abdomen without doing appendicectomy, the worst thing to happen is faecal fistula, and because drainage was kept the faecal matter will come out and general peritonitis can be prevented. It is said the surgeon is never fearless, he fears for the patient, fears for the short comings but never fears for his reputation.

20.4. ACUTE APPENDICITIS TREATED CONSERVATIVELY.

A sub judge daughter studying 8th standard in Palani had lower abdominal pain. The surgeon in Palani examined her and advice emergency surgery for acute appendicitis. The Patient's mother agreed for surgery and the time for surgery was fixed. The mother of the patient informed her husband who was a sub judge in Chennai, about the time of surgery. He told her to take the daughter to Madurai and show her to Dr. Sivalingam, as he has treated many persons in our family. So they arranged a taxi and got admitted in Vadamalayan hospital. I saw the patient in the evening and I had a doubt about the diagnosis and told them that I will see her at 9 PM with abdominal scan and the scan was ordered. I saw the patient at 9.P M. and again I told them I will see her in the morning at 6 Am. when I went to the hospital at 6 A.M. the father also came from Chennai and explained to him that I am not definite about appendicitis. This girl is in pre pubertal stage, some may have abdominal pain periodically before menstruation starts. Because they had confident upon me, they agreed for the waitand see policy and ultimately the patient was discharged without surgery. Later after one month the mother told me that her daughter attained menarche.

20.5. APPENDICECTOMY ON DAY BEFORE DAUGHTERS BETROTHAL.

A lady was admitted for acute appendicitis in vadamalayan hospital. I saw the case and advised emergency appendicectmy. She said next day evening my daughter's engagement is fixed in our house and can I go and attend the function after surgery or can I go attend the function and come back for surgery. I said both are not possible. In that, case I will see you at 5 PM and decide. You will not be discharged today whether I do surgery or not. When I saw her in the evening I decided to do surgery at that time itself. The patient and her husband have agreed for surgery and I did surgery at-5-30 PM. Next day the function was conducted as planned in their house and the whole team came to the hospital to get blessings from the patient. One must understand that in such situation if a lady accepted for surgery means, she was suffering so much from appendicitis pain. Everything went on well, the surgery and the betrothal function and the patient was discharged on 6th post operative day after suture removal.

20.6. LADY HOUSE SURGEON APPENDICECTOMY 10 DAYS BEFORE MARRAIGE.

A lady house surgeon was admitted in our unit on our admission day. I examined her; she had acute appendicitis and the needed surgery. She said her marriage is fixed within 10 days. Her would be, is also a House surgeon and he was with her in the ward. I told them in that case I wait up to 12 mid night. If the pain is reducing with treatment I will treat you conservatively, if not I will do surgery. They agreed. I was on duty on that day. I saw her in the evening and again at mid night. I am not happy with the progress. I told her it is better you get operated now. She said the bridegroom family may cancel the marriage as it is an 'apa sagunam' for marriage. This type of thinking is quite normal in our society. But, the would be bridegroom said you do the surgery, I will convince my parents. So I did the surgery. The Post operative period was uneventful. The bride groom family members came to the hospital and saw her and had discussion and said they have decided to postpone the marriage for 2 months and date of marriage will be fixed after 2 month. I saw her after 6-7 months in the hospital and she said she is pregnant; they have not invited me for the marriage. But I got marriage invitations for her daughter and I attended the marriage at Madurai. These are the cases can be considered as examples that acute appendicitis can occur at any time and at any situation and surgery if indicated, surgery should be done without considering other factors, to save the life or complications of appendicitis. A crucial decision will be needed in such situations.

20.7. PATIENT HAD APPENDICITIS IN MEENAKSHI AMMAN TEMPLE.

A group of people from Usilampatty nearby area were on their way to Ayyappan temple went to Madurai Meenakshi Amman temple. One of them developed acute abdominal pain. Somebody has directed them to my clinic as my clinic is near the temple. I examined the patient. It was a case acute appendicitis and needs emergency surgery. One of them promised that they will go back to Usilampatty and get operated there, and asked me to give Injections for the pain now. The father said Ayyappan will save my son give injections now we will go to the temple. I said why you don't think that Ayyappan has given warning at Madurai where all the facilities are available for treatment and suppose appendicitis occurs during your journey where will you go for treatment. The whole team may suffer. Now your son can be operated at Madurai or in usilampatty. Other people can proceed to Ayyappan temple. They had some discussion for some time. After discussion they said what you said is correct we leave the patient and his father for surgery at Madurai, if something happens in the forest we will be in trouble and the patient's life is at risk. I admitted the patient in Vadamalayan hospital and operated in that night and the patient was discharged without any complications.

20.8. APPENDICULAR ABSCESS.

Though I have treated more cases of appendicular abscess, two cases were more problematic and as a life saving measures I did drainage of appendicular abscess with calculated risk. The first case was admitted in a private hospital in Madurai where Dr.C.Kalidoss goes as consultant. He saw the patient and said that it is a case of appendicular mass; as the general condition of the patient is poor, treat conservatively. Then the owner of that private hospital rang up to me and asked me to see the case. I saw the case. It was an appendicular abscess just pointing out right lumbar region. But his general condition was poor and unless the pus is let out his general condition will not improve.

I told the hospital owner who is a Physician about the condition and unless the pus is let out the patient will not survive.- He said you discuss with Dr.C.Kalidoss. I talked with Dr.Kalidoss and told him the pus can be let out under local and save the patient. Dr. Kalidoss said he will be coming within 30 minutes and asked me to fix the anaesthetist. The anaesthetist is known to the patient and I talked about the patient. He said the patient is unfit for anaesthesia but you do it under local. I said I know the pus has to be let out under local and your help is needed for monitoring the condition during surgery. He agreed. By that time DR.C.K has come. He said you proceed with the case I will assist you. I drained one kidney try full of thick pus under local infiltration with monitoring by the anaesthetist. After 48 hours I saw the patient the temperature was coming down and the patient looked cheerful. After discharge, the patient came to my clinic and thanked me for saving his life. He said he was eagerly waiting for my opinion and when you said can be operated under local even at that critical condition

I was happy that you are going to do something for me and he said I really appreciate your attitude towards the patients in critical condition.

20.9. ACUTE APPENDICITIS IN A JAUNDICED PATIENT. (MEDICAL STUDENT)

Another case was a medical student from Stanley medical college. He is a native of Madurai. He came for vocation to the native place near Madurai. He developed Jaundice and he was under treatment in Intensive Medical Care Unit. He had lower abdominal pain. Prof.C.Raman saw him in I.M.C.U. and said appendicitis and to be treated conservatively. I was surgical registrar at that time (1982-83) and I was called to see him after 2 days. By that time appendicular mass has developed. Once the mass is formed surgery is contraindicated. Because it may be difficult to find out the appendix and the chances of faecal fistula are more. Moreover he has jaundice. So I advised conservative treatment. Appendicular abscess formed within 3 days. I asked Prof.C.R whether the abscess can be drained now. He said it is a highly risky case so it is not advisable. Next day evening the patient's father came to my clinic and told me that people advise me to take my son to Chennai by plane to have a better treatment. I am a teacher my financial position will not permit me to take my son by plane to Chennai. When I discussed with others they directed me to see you and so I have come to see you. Kindly do something for my son. Whatever the complications come we will accept.

Then I told him, I will see him tomorrow at 8-30 AM talk with Dr.C.R and do something for the patient. Next day after seeing the patient, I rang up to Dr.C.R. and told him that the appendicular abscess needs to be drained. He said it is a high risk case you explain to the relatives and do it. I took the case to emergency theatre at 10AM. The chief anaesthetist Dr.Viswanathan himself has come for the case and told me you do it under local and I will monitor the Cardio pulmonary system.

After giving the local field block, I told the chief anaesthetist in a low voice that if the patient dies I will be forced to leave this institution. When I drained two kidney trays full of thick pus I was very happy. The patient was discharged after one week without faecal fistula. He continued the medical course at Stanley medical college. I did not have any contact with him for some time. After 7 or 8 years, he came to colorectal ward with some invitations in his hand. I asked him what happened to you I have not seen you for many years. He said after completion of M.B.B.S., I went to foreign country and now returned and going to start a hospital. I have come here to invite you for the function and I request you to inaugurate the operation theatre and I have printed your name without your consent. I attended the function and declared open the operation theatre. Now that medical centre has developed well as Devaki hospital, CT, Scan, M R I etc.

These two cases are the classical examples that even in desperate condition, if you think the surgery may save the life and the possibility of survival is even less than 10%, surgery should be done. If you don't do the surgery the patient is going to die, why not take a chance to save the life? That is why it is said that a surgeon must have Loin's heart as one of the characters of a surgeon. The other characters are, he must have Ladies Fingers (for gentle Touch), Eagles eye (for good observation), and camel belly to work continuously (surgery) for hours together even without water.

20.10. ACUTE APPENDICITIS WHILE WRITING ENTRANCE EXAMINATION.

A student studying +2 had appendicitis just 2 weeks before the examination. He came to my clinic. I examined him and said you have appendicitis and needs surgery. He said, he has +2 examinations within two weeks and I am interested in engineering and can you postpone the surgery. He also said I am doing my +2 with the help of some social organizations. They promised me to help for my engineering study. I told him I will examine you in the evening and decide. But whatever I say at that time you must accept it. I admitted him in Vadamalayan hospital and started I.V. fluid, antibiotics and ordered for routine investigations for surgery. When I examined him in the evening there was some improvement and so I said I will see him at 9 PM and decide. In the night he was comfortable and so I decided to treat him conservatively so that he could wrights +2 examination. He passed the +2 examination with good marks and told me that he is preparing for the entrance examination after the exam he will come for interval appendicectomy. When he was writing the entrance exam, he had acute abdominal pain and sued down in the examination hall half an hour before the examination is to over. He recovered it consciousness and asked the teachers to admit him in vadamalayan hospital. They took him to Town

Clinic which is nearer to the examination centre. That vadamalayan Town Clinic has been given lease to some other doctor. He told that doctor that surgery should be done only by Dr.Sivalingam. That doctor was my student and called me to see the case. I saw the patient and decided to do appendicectomy immediately because of the clinical findings. As operation theatre was not available in that hospital the patient was transferred to Vadamalayan hospital and within two hours I operated him. Later he came to my clinic and said he has passed the entrance examination with high score and got seat in engineering College.

Ten years later in 1994 he came to my clinic and asked me sir do you remember me, though I am not definite, I asked, it is you who had appendicitis while righting the entrance exam. He was very happy that I remember the incidence and told his name. He said he joined one of the overseas companies and worked in different places and now in one of the islands near Singapore. I told him that I will be attending a conference at Conventional Hall in Singapore in July 1994.

He said he will make arrangements for my stay at Singapore. I told him everything has been made by the conference organizers and the hotel they have not informed me yet. He said I will meet you in Singapore.

Before I start to Singapore, I asked the children to write what are the things I must buy for them in a paper and put it in my suit case. At Singapore when I saw the list almost all are commonly available items which I can buy except my son's list. He asked to buy 10 tape records. I do not know where to buy them. As promised that patient came to Conventional Hall. We had some formal talk he asked me should he buy anything for the children. I gave the list of Tape Records written by my son and told him to buy as much as possible in that list. He asked me to come for shopping and see around the Singapore.

Since I have to present a paper in the Conference I gave him some Singapore dollars and asked him to get the tape records. Surprisingly he bought all tape records written in the list and a head cleaner for tape recorder. My son was very happy and asked me how you bought all the items. I told him that all are bought by a person for whom I have done appendicectomy ten years back in Madurai.

21. GALL BLADDER SURGERY.

21.1. CHOLECYSTECTOMY.

In 1991 two patients were waiting for Gallbladder surgery. When I am going for rounds in Vadamalayan hospital, I asked the first patient whether surgery can be done tomorrow. She said I don't want surgery tomorrow. I asked her why. She said tomorrow is 'astami'. I am surprised to hear because she is a Muslim patient and I asked her will you see all these she said yes. I went to the next patient and asked her whether I can do surgery tomorrow. She said yes you can do. Since she is a Hindu patient I told her tomorrow is 'astami'. She said she will not see all these and family members have come and you operate tomorrow. She had surgery without any problem. After astami and navomi, the Muslim patient was taken to the operation theatre for surgery. There was some difficulty in introducing the endotracheal tube, and finally she developed pulmonary oedema and she was kept in I.C. U. for 2 days. I usually prepare the operation area with antiseptic agent after the anaesthesia is given. So in this case also surgical preparation was not done and the patient was transferred to I.C.U. She was discharged and asked her to come after 2 weeks for surgery. This time the endotracheal tube could be passed without any difficulty and the surgical technique was carried out without any difficulty.

21.2. POST OPERATIVE RESPIRATORY FAILURE.

In 1994 one patient was operated for gall stones in Govt. Rajaji Hospital. The patient was sent to post operative ward. Within five minutes the post operative ward nurse informed us that the patient has some respiratory problems. I asked her to bring the patient to recovery room in operation theatre. By the time I informed the Chief anaesthetist and once the patient arrived, endotracheal tube was passed and other measures for resuscitation of the patient were given. The Chief anaesthetist said let the patient be in recovery room for some time. When our operation list was over, the anaesthetist said the patient can be transferred to post operative ward. I am not satisfied with the condition of the patient and so I asked the anaesthetist to keep some more time in the recovery room. He said the patient has recovered well and can be transferred to post operative ward. I informed the chief anaesthetist, he saw the case and said do not remove the endotracheal tube now and keep the patient in recovery room for some more time. I deputed one house surgeon for bed side duty. I saw the patient at 5-30 PM. The endotracheal tube was removed in my presence and after 30 minutes he was transferred to post operative ward. I saw the case at 9 pm and his respiration was normal.

21.3. CHOLECYSTECTOMY POSTPONED IN THE OPERATION THEATRE.

Mr.Ramasamy from Jakkampatti near Andipatti had gallstones with Cholecystitis (Calculus cholecystitis).He was investigated and posted for surgery.

When I entered the theatre the anaesthetist Dr. Krishnan asked me, are you particular in doing this case today. I asked him why asked the question and I am not particular in doing this case today if you are not satisfied. He said the cardiac monitor shows evidence of ischemia where as the previous E.C.G was normal. I said we will postpone the case today and get the cardiac status assessment by the Cardiologist then we can operate. I talked with the patient in the operation theatre itself. He said whatever you say I will accept. I explained the situation to his wife and other members of the family and they also agreed for further investigations before surgery. These people are known to me for so many years and so there was no problem in post poning the surgery. The Cardiologist examined the patient and did the cardiac investigations, confirmed the ischemic heart disease. He treated the case for 3 months and gave the fitness certificate for surgery, and then cholecystectomy was done.

21.4. LAPAROSCOPIC CHOLECYSTECTOMY IN WORKSHOP.

A surgeon from Selam referred a case of acute Cholecystitis on my admission day. The patient had delivered a baby just 3 months back and had acute attack of cholecystitis. In view of 3 months baby, breast feeding, no relations in Madurai, if I operate by open technique she has to be in the hospital for a minimum of 10 days. At that time the workshop on Laparoscopic surgery was to be conducted on the next day. Dr.Vijayan asked me whether he can operate that case in Laparoscopic work shop. I said yes you can do and I can discharge the case within 2 days. If there is any problem doing Laparoscopic surgery, I can do the surgery by open technique. He wanted me to be in the operation theatre. I said I will be in the auditorium with the delegates and other doctors and if I think that there is a problem during Laparoscopic surgery I will be coming to the theatre. Once the gallbladder was viewed as projected in the screen, I was sure that the gall bladder can be removed without any problems. After the surgery Dr.Vijayan came to the auditorium and thanked me for permitting him to do this case. I said I must thank Dr.Vijayan for doing the surgery for this case because the patient has 3 months old child, which cannot be kept in the hospital because of fear of the child getting hospital infection, now I can discharge her within two days. So it is a mutual help for the patient and the delegates of this Laparoscopic workshop. It was a very good demonstration of Lap Cholecystectomy.

21.5. BARIUM MEAL STUDY?. CHOLEDOCHO DUODENAL FISTULA.

Barium meal Study was done for a patient who had upper abdominal pain. The Radiologist gave the report as choledocho duodenal fistula. But clinically there were no symptoms of recurrent biliary infection. The patient was given soda for the formation of gas in the stomach and X ray abdomen in erect position was taken to see any gas in the biliary system but the gas can not seen in the biliary system. The patient was operated. On the table the common bile duct was carefully examined to find out any biliary fistula. There was duodenal ulcer only. Vagotomy and Posterior gastro Jejunostomy was done. The patient was followed regularly for one year for any recurrent biliary symptoms.

22. BOWEL PERFORATIONS.

22.1. DUODENAL PERFORATION.

22.1.1. PERFORATION IN THE HOSPITAL INPATIENT.

A patient was admitted for acute upper abdominal pain from casualty. On examination he had slight tenderness in right side of epigastrium and no other signs suggestive of perforative peritonitis. X ray abdomen shows no gas under the diaphragm. So the patient was under observation. Next day in regular rounds in the morning the patient was comfortable. I saw the patient during my night rounds at 8-30 PM. There was no complaint from the patient. After one hour PG (Dr. Jayachandran) came for night rounds. At that time the patient had severe abdominal pain and marked tenderness in the right side of epigastrium. He ordered for a X Ray abdomen which showed gas under the diaphragm. He rang up to me and said the findings and said it is perforation. I asked him to prepare the case of surgery, inform the theatre, and the anaesthetist, I will be coming within one hour. When I came to the theatre everything was ready. I asked Dr.Jeyachandren to do the surgery and I assisted him. Post operatively duodenal fistula has formed which was treated conservatively. Later after 6 months Vagotomy and posterior gastrojejunostomy was done for duodenal ulcer. Ian Arid in his book on Companion in Surgery has said the worst place to occur perforation is, perforation occurring in the hospital itself. In his case as myself and PG. regularly doing night rounds and so we were able to find out the perforation, and operated the case immediately. If night rounds were not made when the patient complained of pain abdomen, would have been treated symptomatically till we come for morning round at 8.30 AM.

22.1.2. PG SAID IT IS NOT A CASE OF PERFORATION.

A patient was admitted for acute abdominal pain from casualty. I asked one PG to see the case. He said his findings. Then I examined the patient, it was a case of duodenal ulcer with perforation. He did not accept my diagnosis. I have demonstrated him clinical findings of muscle guarding in the epigastrium and obliteration of Liver dullness. X ray abdomen in erect position showed the gas under the diaphragm. Still he is not convinced about the muscle guarding and gas under the diaphragm for which he said it is the lung shadow below the rib. Now I asked him to operate the case. It was a case of duodenal perforation. He closed the perforation. Unfortunately this patient had duodenal fistula which was treated conservatively. We published a paper on External duodenal fistula in Indian Medical Journal.

22.1.3. DUODENAL PERFORATION IN SITUS INVERSES TOTALIS.

A case of perforation was admitted on our admission day. X ray abdomen showed gas under the diaphragm. I asked the P.G. to do the case. When P.G was doing the surgery, particularly in emergency, I will be in the operation theatre sitting on a revolving stool. The PG said he could not find out the duodenum and he asked my help. I asked the assistant to lift up the retractor so that I can see the site. He put the retractor and lifted up the right costal margin easily. I said he careful the liver should not be damaged. As I had the doubt, I asked them to look for the liver. The liver was not on the right side and it was on left side. Now I joined with operating team. When the stomach and intestines were examined, it was a case of Situs Inverses. The duodenum was on the left side with perforation. The perforation was closed and the Abdomen was closed with a drain. After surgery we reviewed the X ray abdomen the side marking was not done in the X ray. The anaesthetist auscultated the chest for heart position and said the heart is on the right side of the chest.

The anaesthetist missed the Dexio Cardia during pre anaesthetics chest examination. Here I remember the Phrase given in Boyd Pathology Book that our eyes do not see what our mind does not know. In this case our PG. could not make out the Mal rotation and the anaesthetist could not make out the Dexio Cardia. So we have missed ' Situs Inverses Totalise. I took one postoperative X-ray abdomen with proper marking of the side in X-ray plate. When showed the post operative X ray to other unit PGs some of them gave the correct answer and some said the side marking on the X Ray is wrong. I asked the people to auscultate the chest of the patient to find out the Dexio Cardia. Here again I told them before you find fault with others check yourself, are you correct? This case was presented in Clinical Society meeting.

22.1.4. DUODENAL PERFORATION IN VADAMALAYAN HOSPITAL.

I just finished an operation and writing operation notes in Vadamalayan hospital, a lady patient came by climbing the steps and told me she heard a loud sound in her abdomen one hour earlier and after that she has upper abdominal pain. As she was talking with me she fell down due to pain. I examined her and it was a case of perforative peritonitis. Another surgeon was operating in the theatre. I asked the anaesthetist be ready for a case of perforation. Investigations were done in the mean time and l.V fluids were started and other preoperative preparations were done. She was living near Vadamalayan hospital so she came with her husband a little earlier after the acute attack. Ian Arid said in duodenal perforation the patient can say the exact time when the perforation has occurred as in this case. She was operated within two hours of the incidence. The duodenal perforation was closed. After suture removal the patient had burst abdomen which was sutured under local. Her husband said he cannot spend money and he left her in the hospital and never came back. I asked her to go to GRH for further treatment but she refused. So she was treated with sample antibiotics and vitamins and her general condition was deteriorated and her mother was the only person by the side of the patient and the patient died. Within one month of the death of the patient, her husband was distributing sweets to vadamalayan hospital staffs. When asked why you are giving sweets to everybody he told them that he got married to a lady doctor. It seems he was waiting the patient to die for the second marriage.

22.1.5. DUODENAL PERFORATION IN AN AYYAPPAN DEVOTEE.

A group of peoples after visiting Ayyappan temple went to Meenakshi Amman temple. While they are going around the temple inside one of them had severe abdominal pain and he was taken to Dr.Chelliah clinic. He took X ray abdomen which showed gas under the diaphragm. He referred the case to me. It was a case of perforative peritonitis and admitted in Vadamalayan hospital. I told the people who accompany him that the patient needs an emergency surgery. They said they are returning from Ayyappan temple in a van and they have spent all the money, now you give him some injection and we will take him to Theni for treatment there. I told them it is dangerous to continue the journey. Surgery should be done as early as possible. Then they said you do the surgery and we will bring money tomorrow. I asked them at least one person must stay with the patient. His brother in law agreed to stay with him. I told the nurse to look after the attender; I will look after the patient. Surgery was done in that night itself; it was perforation of duodenal ulcer. The perforation was closed. The patient's wife came two days later. I told her that we were expecting you yesterday itself but you have come today only. She said they told me in the night and I made arrangements for the money and came now. The tension is my mind was relieved. The post operative period was smooth and the patient was discharged without any complications. In this case the patient and the relatives believed me and I believed them and God saved the patient.

22.1.6. DUODENAL PERFORATION WITH PERIGASTRIC ABSCESS.

A case was admitted as carcinoma of stomach with epigastric mass. In the operation table the mass was in the para duodenal area and the stomach was normal. When the mass was mobilised, the tissues were friable due to inflammatory tissue. Diagnostic aspiration was done and thick puss was aspirated and sent for bacteriological culture. The abscess cavity was opened and about 50 cc of thick puss was let out. The abscess wall was taken for biopsy and abscess cavity was drained. The wound was closed with corrugators drain. Heavy antibiotic was given. Sutures were removed and the patient was discharged.

He came to our review clinic after 4 or 5 months with another patient and I could not recognize him. One of the PGs said that he is our old patient with peri gastric abscess. The patient has not brought the old records and asked him which month he was operated, He told the month and date. I sent the PG to record room to collect the old case sheet and found out what the P.G said was correct. In those days with limited investigations, when the patient needed surgery, depending upon the clinical findings it was done. Depending upon the operative findings the diagnosis may be different. That is why it is said the abdomen is a Temple of Surprise or a Magic Box. Now with modern investigations, the abdomen is neither a Magic Box nor Temple of surprise. Everything must be definite before you take up the case for surgery. Now place of explorative laparotomy has a very limited place.

22.1.7. A CASE OF GAS UNDER THE DIAPHRAGM.

When I was on duty one case was referred to GRH by my teacher as bowel perforation. He has taken X-ray abdomen which showed gas under the diaphragm. Clinically there was no suspicion of peritonitis. She was treated by naso gastric aspiration, IV fluids and antibiotics. I reviewed her back at 7 pm and even now the abdomen was soft and there is no evidence of peritonitis. Blood pressure, pulse rate and temperature were normal. Since the case was referred by my teacher I did not want to miss the diagnosis. I told my PGs that I am going to review at12.30 Am and decide. I talked with the patient as I am seeing her for the first time. As I am eliciting her history of her marital status, she told that she was married 5 years back and has no child. I asked her have you seen any doctor for not having child. She said she had consulted Dr.Sabitha, gynaecologist in Madurai. She tested me by pushing air into the vagina. Now we know that she had done tube test where air is pushed in to the uterus to find out the patency of Fallopian tube. The test was done two days earlier. So radio logically there was air under the diaphragm and clinically there was no evidence of peritonitis. Now I asked the nurse to remove the nasogastric tube, stop I V. fluid and allow the patient to take fluids orally. During the morning rounds she was normal and same day she was discharged. My chief used to say that we treat the patient and not the X ray. This case proved his statement

22.2. ILEAL PERFORATION.

22.2.1. ENTERIC PERFORATION.

One of our PG students said he has not seen an enteric perforation go alive from the hospital. On that day we had an enteric perforation in a girl. I asked that PG do that case and I assisted him. The perforation in the ileum was closed. The sutures were removed and the patient was to be discharged next day. But the patient developed bursts abdomen which was sutured under local. After one year she came for incisional hernia which was operated by me and the PG who did the closure of the perforation assisted me. The patient was discharged after suture removal. Now I told the PG if we have not operated her for enteric perforation she could have died. That is why our chief, Dr.S.Shanmugam used to say that we want to have a living problem than death certainty. After one year the mother of the girl asked me whether her daughter can get married. I said yes, but wait for another one year.

22.2.2. ENTERIC PERFORATION MR. THANGAVELU.

Mr.Thangavelu, a case of enteric perforation closure was done under general anaesthesia. I was told that the chief anaesthetist Dr.Srinivasan had asked the duty anaesthesiologist why you gave anaesthesia for a case of enteric perforation, when there is 100% mortality in surgery. Even when the surgeon asks you could have refused to give anaesthesia. Let him do under local or let him do bilateral flank drain under local. Next day I showed the Journals to the Chief anaesthetist where articles have come which say surgical intervention can save life in enteric perforations. After suture removal I showed the case to him and said the patient is to be discharged today. I think he is convinced because subsequent cases of enteric perforations were operated under general anaesthesia in our unit. I showed three cases of enteric perforation operated in our unit to the chief anaesthetist and I said the present trend is close the ileal perforation and give peritoneal wash and close the abdomen with a drain. Of course the post operative complications like faecal fistula, wound infections and burst abdomen can occur. PeristonN, a detoxicating agent, manufactured by Bayer Company, was used for the first time in this case. Sutures are removed on the tenth post operative day. That night when I came for night rounds, he had burst abdomen and it was sutured under local. After two days when I was making morning regular ward rounds the patient behaved a little indifferently and I got annoyed and a slapped on his face and preceded the ward rounds. After I finished all my ward works at 1:45 PM the nurse said that the patient Thangavel wanted to talk with you personally. I asked him to come. When he came he said my brother in law asked me Rs 250 to give you. I said he is not of that type. He said he has made arrangement for that. So I gave the money on that night when you operated me second time. Now I know that he has taken that money. I will ask him when he comes in the evening. But his brother in law never came after that incidence. The patient was discharged after suture removal.

22.2.3. MASTER KAMARAJ. A CASE OF ENTERIC PERFORATION.

Twelve years Kamaraj was operated to ileal perforation due to Typhoid fever. I advised Periston N during my rounds. As it is not available in the hospital his mother has to buy outside. Just before I leave the ward, the nurse asked me sir is it absolutely necessary to buy Periston N, because the patient's mother is a widow and poor. I said it is better to give all injections.

If it is not possible we treat will the available drugs in the hospital. It seems the nurse explained the mother and she sold one large size brass pot and got the money and bought Periston N. Sutures were removed on the tenth day. One doctor who is planning to go to USA wanted to have some exposure to surgical cases so he joined as senior house surgeon in our unit. He used to be in the ward during my night rounds. That night the patient Kamaraj was sleeping. There was some blood staining in the dressing. I told that senior house surgeon that we have removed the sutures today morning and now the dressing is blood stained, the wound must be inspected though the patient is sleeping. I removed the dressing there was bursts abdomen. I wake up the boy and said the internal sutures have given away and needs to be sutured, is there anybody with you. He said my brother is here on the floor, you ask him. He was younger than the patient, around ten years, and told him your brother needs immediate surgery. We cannot wait till other person comes. He said yes you can do surgery. We took him to operation theatre and sutured the wound. The patient was discharged on the 10th day of secondary suturing. Both cases were presented in the Clinical Society meeting and we stressed the use of Periston N in these cases and surgical closure of the enteric perforation to save the life. Later Periston N was available in GRH.

22.2.4. MULTIPLE ENTERIC PERFORATIONS VELAYUTHAM.

Mr.Velayutham from Sivarakkotai was operated for enteric perforation. There were three perforations of about 5 CM apart each. All the perforations were sutured and abdomen was closed with a drain. He developed burst abdomen which was sutured. Faecal fistula occurred thrown the abdominal wound. Two abdominal sutures were removed on the 3rd day for effective drainage; the intestinal mucosa was seen in the abdominal wound. After the general condition improved to some extent, he was taken for surgery. The ileum was adherent to the abdominal wound with fistula segment. The adhesions are released and the defect in the ileum was closed. He went home without any further complications.

After many years when I was making rounds in vadamalayan hospital, one person was following me and I asked what he wants. He said his name is Velayutham. Then asked him are you from Sivarakotai? He was very happy when I said his village name, immediately I recognized him and asked about him. He said he is working in Chennai, married and has one child; he has come to see his mother who was admitted for Cardiac problems this hospital. I asked him to show his abdomen and operated scar. Then I told his history to my nurse. I was very happy to see him after many years, well settled in life.

On those days we use chromic catgut for abdominal closure which is absorbable and may give way when infection is present. So the wound complications like bust abdomen and incisional hernia were common occurrence.

Now we use non absorbable Prolene for abdominal closure. So these complications are reduced. More over the incidence of enteric perforation is markedly reduced.

22.3. SIGMOID COLON PERFORATION.

22.3.1.

When I started the Colorectal Department in 1982 December I was trying to get instruments for the department. After one year I got one old type of rigid Sigmoidoscope, transferred from main operation theatre. In that the light is in the distal end of the scope. When Sigmoidoscopic biopsy is needed we have to remove the light from the scope and take biopsy blindly. I had three cases of Sigmoid Perforation among those who had sigmoidoscopic biopsy within a period of four months of its use.

The First case, I made out the perforation on the next day morning 8.30 AM itself when the patient came to see me who had sigmoidoscopic biopsy on the previous day. I advised admission and emergency surgery. The patient wanted the surgery to be done by a particular surgeon. I talked with the assistant of that unit and the Patient was admitted in that unit and surgery was fixed at l I AM. Then it was postponed to 2 PM and again to 6 P M and at last surgery was done at 10 PM about 13 hours after diagnosis of colonic perforation was made. The patient died within 24 hours of surgery.

The Second case was Mr. Regupathy Medical college office staff. He had pain in left lower abdomen after Sigmoidoscopy. He was admitted for observation. X ray abdomen showed no gas under the diaphragm. When I went for night rounds the duty assistant told me that Mr Ragupathy has lower abdominal pain, clinically the abdomen is normal. I saw the patient. There was clinical evidence of Peritonitis. I told the patient what has happened and he needs immediate surgery. He agreed for surgery. I operated the patient in the night itself within one hour of diagnosis. He was discharged without any complication.

The 3rd case was operated by Dr.Lakshmana Perumal on his duty day for perforation following sigmoidoscopic biopsy on the same night and the patient was transferred to colorectal ward. This patient also went home without any complications. There were so many remarks and comments about the Perforation following sigmoidoscopy among the assistants in surgical side. In a way criticisms actually help you to work on the path of perfection. Large bowel perforation must be operated as early as possible once the diagnosis is made. After the first case of perforation following sigmoidoscopy, I was quite reluctant to do sigmoidoscopy. But I was forced to do the other two cases. I stopped doing Sigmoidoscopy and sent a letter for purchase of Sigmoidoscope with Cold light source and Biopsy forceps, and got within 2 months and started doing sigmoidoscopic biopsy and about 5-6 cases were done on one out patient day. We had 3 days OP in a week and one operation day in a week.

About 40 cases were been seen on one out patient day and a minimum of 16 cases were operated including both major and minor cases in one operation day.

23. BOWEL OBSTRUCTION.

23.1. GASTRIC OUTLET OBSTRUCTION.

23.1.1. CONGENITAL PYLORIC STENOSIS.

A three month old child was brought to Virudunagar Hospital for vomiting immediately after feeding. The Paediatrician asked me to see the case. It was a case of Congenital Pyloric Stenosis and I have palpated the mass in the right side of epigastrium while examining the baby in the first time itself. I told the mother the child needs surgery; I will give a letter to GRH Madurai and take the Child to Madurai. She and her husband wers field labourers and have two other Children. She said she cannot go to Madurai leaving those children. You are doing surgery for many people; like that you operate my child also. If you are not doing surgery, whatever happens to the child let it happen and I will not go to Madurai. I have worked in Paediatric surgery department for one year as assistant surgeon in GRH Madurai and I have done 3 cases of Pyloric Stenosis. Considering their financial problem and family situations, I agreed to take up the case for surgery. I informed the DMO and operated the child. The Baby was discharged in 3 days. The vomiting has stopped. I first wanted to refer the case to Madurai because if complications occur during surgery and if the child dies, I have to face difficult situation. Now the mother says even if the baby dies she will not go to Madurai because of other children. Situation like this we have to take a calculated risk to operate. That is why it was said that the surgeon is never fearless, he fears for the patient, fears for the short coming during surgery, but never fears for his reputation.

23.1.2. PATIENT ATE 3 ORANGES IN FIRST P.O. day.

A patient came to me with chronic duodenal ulcer with obstruction. Vagotomy and gastrojejunostomy was done at Vadamalayan hospital. The Patient had taken three kamala oranges as such. I treated him conservatively with nothing by mouth and I.V. fluids. The patient was carefully watched for stoma obstruction. On the 5th post operative day he passed motion. Then only he was permitted to take orally and fortunately he become alright and discharged after suture removal. Same thing happened in GRH. The patient from Kodailkanal took oranges in the 3rd post operative day and he was also treated conservatively.

23.1.3. POSTERIOR GASTROJEJUNOSTOMY IN VIRUDUNAGAR HOSPITAL.

When I am working in Virudunagar Headquarter Hospital I operated a case of chronic duodenal ulcer with obstruction. Vagotomy and Posterior gastrojejunostomy was done. After suture removal I discharged the patient and advised him not go for work for one month and come after ten days for review. He said he is alone and coming from a village about 30 KM away from here. Unless I go for the work as a casual labourer I will not get anything for my food and nobody is there to look after me. Then I told the nurse don't discharge him and keep him in the ward for hospital food. He was very happy and he gained weight more than my expectation and I asked the nurse how he gained weight. She said that other patient's attenders also gave food for him. After one month the patient was discharged and advised to go for light works for some times.

23.1.4. P.G.J. DONE UNDER LOCAL.

Sometimes the anaesthetists will not asses the case for anaesthesia, because of dehydration, malnutrition, and electrolyte imbalance. As the patient has persistent vomiting after taking anything due to duodenal obstruction this is no chance of correcting the dehydration and other parameters of Biochemical values. If the duodenal obstruction is relived by doing gastro jejunostomy the patient will recover from all these defects. So in these cases I took calculated risk, inform the relatives and operate under local field block. I have operated 15 cases under local. One patient developed Cardiac arrest and one patient developed respiratory arrest. Both patients were resuscitated by the anaesthetist. One of the P.G. in anaesthesia department (Dr.Valavanthan Rathinam) who was my senior in medical college selected Central Venus Pressure recording in severely dehydrated patients operated under general anaesthesia as his dissertation topic. Maximum number of cases were done in that trail, from our unit. So during trial period all non assessed cases of duodenal obstruction were posted for surgery and our

PG will inform Dr.Valavathan Rathinam on the previous day. Usually these patients gain weight of 1 kg after surgery; where as other patients loose 1 kg in post operative period.

23.1.5. GASTRIC OUTLET OBSTRUCTION WITH CARDIAC DISEASE.

A case was referred as gastric out let obstruction with visible gastric peristalsis from medial side and they have also mentioned no cardiac disease. The patient was admitted and investigated and sent to medical side for E.C.G opinion for the purpose of anaesthetic assessment. Their opinion was mitral valvular disease and the patient is fit for surgery as far as the cardiac condition is concerned. The patient was brought buy a house surgeon Arunagiredayalan. After anaesthetic assessment, the patient was posted for surgery and P.G.J. was done. On the second post operative day patient was cyanosed and had breathing problem. Now I sent a reference to medical side to call over to post operative ward to see the patient. The physician saw the case and wrote in the case sheet as cyanotic heart disease and advised some medicines which were given to the patient and the patient died on the 4th post operative day. On the following day the physician made some drastic comments about the treatment and said the patient would have lived for another 2 to 3 months with vomiting, but they killed him by doing surgery. This news came to me. I collected the case sheet and went to the medical ward to show that the patient was referred from medical O.P. and has written as no cardiac condition. Before anaesthetic assessment I got medical opinion with E.C.G. and X-ray chest, now they have written as mitral stenosis without failure and fit for surgery as far as cardiac condition is concerned. In the 2nd post operative day, the patient was referred from post operative ward to medical side and the physician had written as cyanotic heart disease. We have not done the surgery without getting preoperative fitness from the physician. How can he say that we have killed the patient by doing surgery? His assistant Dr Alagappan said you know that sometimes he will talk some loose talk. Like that he talked in this case without knowing the condition he has given fitness certificate for surgery as far as the cardiac condition, I will tell him later. Now you please go to your ward. I had confident that Dr Alagappan would have told the physician about this case.

23.1.6. DUODENAL ILEUS.

A 25 years male was admitted as duodenal ulcer with obstruction. On examination the patient was dehydrated and anaemic. The stomach was markedly dilated with VGP occupying the whole of the upper abdomen extending down to the level of umbilicus, no mass was palpable. When I asked the patient how long he has these symptoms. The patient said he had abdominal pain on and off and occasional vomiting, for the fast one year the vomiting was severe. He was investigated for surgery. The blood Bio chemistry was corrected to the optimum level. Stomach wash was given to wash out the stagnant food particles in the stomach. Dehydration was corrected well with I.V fluids and the patient was permitted to take only plain water and tender coconut. At the optimal level of blood biochemistry parameters and Hb level, the patient was posted for surgery. On opening the abdomen, the stomach was found markedly dilated occupying the whole upper abdomen. The duodenum also found dilated up to the 3rd part. Beyond the duodeno jejunal junction, the small intestine is found contracted and no pathology could be made out. When the duodenum was traced down it abruptly ends as narrowing where a thick fibrous band just proximal to the duodeno jejunal junction causing stenosis of the duodenum and proximal dilatation. As the stomach is loaded with fluid I asked the anaesthetist to apply suction to the neso gastric tube and I did repeated manipulation of the tip of the neso gastric tube. After completely sucked the fluid in the stomach, the stomach and duodenum was palpated for any pathology and no pathology could be made out. In view of the patient general condition and his socio economical status, it was decided to do simple procedure like posterior gastro jejunal anatomises. Somebody in our team suggested duodeno jejunostomy. I told the possibility of anastomotic leak is more common in that procedure. If the leak occurs it will be very difficult to manage. So let us be happy with gastrojejunostomy with a little wider stoma giving allowance for the dilated stomach becomes normal. So we did PGJ with wide stoma. Patient had two units of blood during surgery. Human albumin and IV amino acids were given in the post operative period. He had recovered well and discharged with advice to come for review after one month. This case was presented in Clinical Society meeting. One of our assistant presented the case. He stopped presentation after describing the operative findings, and said further presentation will the made by my chief. I said I was just thinking how to proceed, can anyone give suggestion for me. The head of the department of surgery said it is advisable to proceed with duodeno jejunostomy.

I said I did gastrojejunostomy. Now all professors started to objecting the procedure, infects one person said you have done wrong procedure. After hearing all commends I told that, I have not done the wrong procedure, I can show references that PGJ can be done for duodenal ileus. And another point patient's general condition has markedly improved after surgery which you can confirm by seeing the patient here now. If I did Duodeno jejunostomy there is every chances of anastomotic leak. Even now we have done in a compromised condition of the patient. I don't want my patient to go for the complications of Duodeno Jejunostomy and I am not wrong in this case. Then the chairman of the meeting who is also a surgeon said if you have reference please show it. I told him that I never expected such objection in this procedure so I have not brought the reference, I will show in the next meeting. In the next meeting I brought the reference and showed American Text Book of Surgery which quoted that out of 100 cases of duodenal Ileus, 40 cases had PGJ and 60 cases had Duodeno Jejunostomy. The audience particularly the P-G flapped their hands because they know this type of management and only the seniors are not aware of that. A person, who never made mistake, never tried anything new. The seniors are contented with the knowledge obtained and they do not advocate the new methods. Though the PGJ is not a new technique, they are not aware that it can be adapted to duodenal ileus; more over Duodenal ileus is not a common condition in adults.

23.1.7. ACUTE DILATATION OF THE STOMACH.

A case was admitted as volulus of sigmoid colon. X-ray showed dilated bowel up to pelvis. Emergency surgery was done. There was a huge dilated stomach with residual food in the dilated stomach. The large intestines including the sigmoid colon were normal. Decompression of the stomach through nasogastric tube could not be done because of residual food. So a gastrostomy in the anterior wall of the stomach was done, though which all the residual food and fluids were removed by using large size suction tube. A gastric wash was done. The anterior gastrostomy wound was closed and PGJ was done. The patient has recovered and discharged after suture removal. In this instance, I can quote one statement, ' you can be confident in your diagnosis but should not be over confident. In this case, with over confident the diagnosis of volvulus sigmoid was made and it was wrong. But the decision for surgery was correct.

This patient was admitted after 6 months as acute appendicitis in some other unit and referred to our unit for takeover. We transferred his case to our ward. X ray abdomen showed multiple fluid levels in the intestine. He was prepared for emergency surgery.

There were multiple adhesions with gangrene of the ileum. Adhesions were released and the gangrenous segment of ileum was excised and end to end anatomises was done.

23.2. JEJUNAL OBSTRUCTION.

23.2.1. LEOMYOMA OF JEJUNUM WITH L.G.I BLEEDING.

A 35 years female patient was admitted for lower gastro intestinal bleeding, intestinal borborgmy with anaemia. Clinically no mass was palpable in the abdomen. Rectal examination and Sigmoidoscopy showed evidence of bleeding from above the level of Sigmoidoscope. Upper G.I. endoscopy was normal. M.R.I angiogram was done on 15.8.2006 which revealed a vascular tumour in jejunum. Patient had seven units of blood and operated. There was a mass palpable in the Jejunum about 20 cm from duodeno jejunal junction with proximal dilatation. The segment of tumour bearing jejunum was resected and intestinal continuity was established. The biopsy report was Leomyoma of jejunum. In postoperative period the patient had one unit of blood and other supportive therapy. She was discharged after suture removal.

23.2.2. JEJUNAL STRICTURES WITH PERFORATION.

A patient was admitted from casualty for perforative peritonitis. On examination there was tenderness in the umbilical region, no mass was palpable, no liver dullness obliteration and no free fluid in the abdomen. X-ray abdomen shows no gas under the diaphragm and no fluid level. The patient was put on conservative treatment. The patient was reviewed after two hours. There was increase of 2.5cm in abdominal girth and the abdominal pain also increased. So surgery was done. There were two strictures in the jejunum 5 cm apart with perforation in the proximal stricture site. Resection of strictures bearing jejunal segment was done and the specimen sent for Biopsy. The Biopsy report was tuberculus strictures. X-ray chest was taken; there was no evidence of active or healed pulmonary tuberculosis or mediastinal node enlargement. The patient was treated with anti-tuberculosis drugs. Later when referred the book we found that tuberculus stricture with perforation may not show gas under the diaphragm. The patient was readmitted for incision hernia repair.

23.3. ILEAL OBSTRUCTION.

23.3.1. INTUSSUSCEPTION OF MECKEL'S DIVERTICULAM.

Mr. Manickam was admitted through casualty as intussusceptions. The mass palpated in the lower abdomen with classical features of intussusceptions, mass becomes hard when acute abdominal pain occurs. For teaching purposes Ba. Enema was ordered. Everybody in our team said it is ileocolic intussusceptions. I was of opinion that it is Meckel's diverticular intussusceptions, But the P.G. did not convinced. When our chief came for night rounds he saw the Ba Enema and asked everybody what they think and they said it is ileocolic type. He then asked me, I said it is Meckel's intussusceptions and explained my findings. Then the chief said you take this case as emergency and after opening the abdomen inform me, I will come. I asked the P.G. to open the abdomen. After opening the abdomen he called me and said it is ileo ileal type. Chief was informed; he said proceed with the surgery. So I also joined the operating team and did resection of the mass and ileal end to end anatomises was done. I asked the P. G. to cut open the mass and after opening the P. G. said it is Meckel's diverticulam.

Next day the Ba. Enema was shown to the Chief Radiologist. He said it is meckel's intussusceptions and asked me whether was operated. I said yes and your statement is correct. The x ray and the resected specimen were kept in International College of Surgeons Conference at Madurai and a paper was presented later.

23.3.2. SMALL INTESTINAL VOLVULUS FOLLOWING APPENDICECTOMY.

A case of acute appendicitis, with classical symptoms and clinical findings was admitted in Vadamalayan hospital and emergency appendicectomy was done. On the fifth post operative day, the patient developed severe abdominal pain and vomiting. The abdomen was found distended. X ray abdomen showed distended small intestine. The abdominal distension was gradually increasing. So it was decided to operate. I explained the patient and his relatives the need for surgery and they agreed. Dr.Padmalakshmi was the anaesthetist. Once I opened the abdomen, I found that the whole small intestine was in a state of compromised blood supply and distended. I asked the anaesthetist stop nitrous oxide and give 100 % oxygen. I followed the mesentery of small intestine, and there was volvulus all the root of the mesentery and untwisting of the mesentery was done very carefully without producing any traction in the pedicle of the mesentery and mesenteric vessels. Once the derotation was done the normal colour of the intestine regained slowly. When examined the cause for the rotation, the proximal ileum was adherent to the raw area of the appendicular pedicle resulting in twisting in the mesentery. The anaesthetists appreciated my approach to solve the problem. This was possible because my Anatomy knowledge which I gained when I worked as Tutor in Anatomy at Tirunelveli Medical College in 1966 to 1968. The patient recovered from anaesthesia. After one year the parents came and asked whether he can get married. I said yes, he can, and I attended his marriage.

23.3.3. ILEO SIGMOID KNOTTING.

A patient was admitted for volvulus sigmoid. Clinically and Radio logically it was Confirmed. After correcting the dehydration the patient was taken for emergency surgery. Surgery was started by P.G. and he called me and said the sigmoid is gangrenous. So I also washed and joined the team. When I examined I found the small bowel is also gangrenous. Really I do not know the condition in which both small bowel and sigmoid colon gangrene occur. As the gangrenous part has to be removed resection of gangrenous small bowel and sigmoid colon was done. The distal end of the sigmoid colon was sutured (Hartman's procedure). The proximal end was brought out as colostomy. Next day I discussed about the case with one of the senior assistant surgeons, he said it is a case of ileo sigmoid knotting or double volvulus and the operation which you have done is correct. Then I studied about this condition in the journal.

When I reviewed the X ray afterwards, the classical finding of Ileo sigmoid Knotting as described in the Journal was present. That is why it is said our eyes do not see what our mind does not know. The patient was readmitted for colostomy closure. After some years another case was admitted and we are able to diagnose Ileo sigmoid Knotting preoperatively with X ray findings.

23.3.4. INTESTINAL OBSTRUCTION DUE TO ROUND WORM INFESTATION.

A twelve year boy was admitted for intestinal obstruction. When I palpated the abdomen, a doubtful mass was palpated and the obstruction was not complete. So I did Ba enema thinking that it is a case of intussusceptions. When the patient was asked to pass the motion for post evacuation X ray he passed two round worms and the post evacuation film showed multiple round worms. I gave anti helmenthetic tablets and he started passing the round worms. I gave a stick to the patient to count the worms each time he passes motion. He passed worms even after 24 hours of tablets. When I go the DAS quarters people asked me what is the score now Ultimately he passed 864 worms and he come alright. I gave Antihelmenthetic tablets to all the family members. I wanted to publish the case in the Journal and asked Dr.T.DoraiRajan, the Paediatric surgeon how many round worms you have seen, passed by a patient on your practice. He said, why, a Bucket full of worms. So I have not sent the paper for publication. I presented the case in the Clinical Society meeting. After 4 or 5 years the mother of the boy met me in the hospital and said all the members in her family are doing well. I was very happy to hear that. I recollected my memory how scabies was eradicated in a hostel when I was doing my SPM posting at Palamedu in 1966.

23.4. LARGE BOWEL OBSTRUCTION.

23.4.1. DIAGNOSED AS VOLVULUS BUT IT WAS CANCER RECTUM.

Mr.Viswanathan was admitted through casualty as large bowel obstruction. X ray showed dilated pelvic colon, descending colon, and transverse colon. On rectal examination no growth was palpable. Laparotomy was done. The large intestine was markedly dilated. When I traced down, there was a growth in the recto sigmoid region which was responsible for the obstruction. Pelvic colostomy was done and biopsy was taken from the growth. The biopsy report was well differentiated adeno carcinoma. The patient was informed about the biopsy report and told him that you need another operation. The second operation was done one month later. There were milliary nodules on the peritoneum and over the small bowel. Biopsy was taken from the peritoneal nodules. The biopsy report came as foreign body granuloma. On those days autoclaved reusable gloves with Salk powder were being used. Because 3 to 4 doctors including P.G. palpated the growth, the stalk powder spread in the peritoneum and small bowel serous layer which is responsible for the granuloma formation. The patient was given available anti mitotic drug (endoxon). There was no progress and the patient died.

23.4.2. LARGE BOWEL OBSTRUCTION DUE TO FECAL IMPACTION.

When I was the casualty medical officer in Govt. Erskine hospital (now Rajaji Hospital) in 1971, a patient came with evidence of large bowel obstruction. I did rectal examination. The rectum was loaded with hard faecal mass with some indentation. Through proctoscope a small bit was taken and examined, there were hairs in the faecal matter. The faecal matter was removed with sponge holding forceps to some extend and soap and water enema was given in the casualty itself and he passed large quantity of hard faecal mass with hairs and the obstruction got relieved. I asked the patient how hair comes in the faces; he said lamp head was cooked in his house 2 days back probably, the hairs were not removed properly. I asked him whether he needs admission. He said now I am relieved from the suffering and so admission is not required. I prescribed liquid paraffin (only available laxative at that time) and advised the patient to come to the hospital if pain comes.

23.4.3. VOLULUS SIGMOID WITH POOR GENERAL CONDITION.

A 55 years man was admitted for volvulus sigmoid. When I examined the case it was volvulus with suspicions of gangrene. The patient was in peripheral shock with tachycardia, low B. P, with dehydration. Catheterization was done only a few CC of urine came. I thought it is a high risk case and he is not fit for any type of anaesthesia. So I asked the nurse put the patient on DIL and explained the patient's condition to one of the male attendee who was present. But regular treatment like I.V fluid, antibiotics were started and Blood was sent for laboratory tests. Now one girl of about 20 years came to me and said she is the daughter of that patient, her marriage was fixed in next month, and she is working in a metal shop near my consulting room. I thought without Surgery the patient will die and her marriage may be cancelled, and I told the PG let us try the luck of that girl. By taking risk you are going to lose less. But not taking risk you are going to lose more. I explained her that table death may occur. In spite that if you agree I will do the surgery. She said whatever happens I agree for the surgery for my father. Now I told my team that start one more I.V drip and let the drips flow fast and at least a total of 1.5 litres of fluid must flow within one hour and the urine output must be a minimum of 5Occ within that time. As directed I.V. fluids were given and the urine output was 6occ I rushed the patient to the operation theatre, and told the anaesthetists, you please have a look of that girl who is the daughter of this patient, I will let you know later and now you start the case. Regular formalities of writing in the case sheet and mention about the anaesthetic risks can he done when the surgery is going on. I take the responsibility if anything happens to patient. I have already explained to the patient's daughter about table death. Dr.Prema, the senior anaesthetist agreed and gave anaesthesia. As suspected, it was a case of volvulus sigmoid with gangrene. The gangrenous bowel was excised, pelvic colostomy and closure of the distal end (Hartman's Procedure) and done. The patient has recovered from anaesthesia. I told the relatives it is better to postpone the marriage for 2 to 3 months as the patient needs one more operation. The patient had a little stormy post operative period but became completely alright. After two months, the colostomy was closed. I was invited for the marriage of his daughter and I attended the marriage.

Situation like this we must explain well about the condition of the patient, the necessity of surgery and the risk factors. If the patient and the relatives understand the need of surgery and the risk factors, will definitely accept the surgery if they know there is no other go. On those days whatever we say, the patients accept. Nowadays will it be possible? I doubt about it:

23.4.4. VOLVULUS SIGMOID. MY LIFE IS IN THAT TOOTH.

Mr.Baladyan was admitted for volvulus Sigmoid. Flatus tube was passed and large quantity of gas came out and his symptoms are relieved. Abdomen distension was also markedly reduced. We have decided to do elective surgery. Anaesthetist wanted shacking tooth to the removed before surgery. The patient was referred to the dental department for extraction of shacking tooth. He refused for the extraction of the tooth because he believed his life is in that tooth and absconded in the evening. After 3 month he was admitted in the evening through the casualty. When the patient was wheeling to ward 218 he said, again to the same ward. I was not aware of that. When I am examining, all the time he turned his face to other side and answered the questions. I turn his face towards me and asked are you Baladyan? Now the stretcher bearer said, while coming to the ward he said why to the same ward. Now the tooth which was shacking had already fallen. When I said about the surgery he agreed and he was operated electively in the next operation day.

24. ANAL PROBLEMS.

24.1. PILES.

24.1.1. LOWER G.I. BLEEDING AFTER PILES SURGERY.

A Paediatrician brought his brother in law for my consultation for bleeding per rectum. The patient has prolapsing piles and advised Surgery. After investigations surgery was done and the patient was discharged with an advice of review after one week. On the 3rd day after discharge the Paediatrician rang up to me and said his brother in law is having bleeding per anus. I asked him to bring the patient to Vadamalayan hospital and inform me after arrival, because the patient has to come from usilampatty area. When the patient came, I examined him; dark coloured blood was coming from above the operated site. I did proctoscopy and sigmoidoscopy, the dark altered blood was coming from above the level of 25cm from anal verge. So Ryle's tube was passed to find out whether the bleeding is from stomach. Some streaks of blood were aspirated. Now I asked the patient whether he has taken any medicine other than what I have advised. I used to prescribe only laxative after surgery. He said after going home, he had pain in the operated area and consulted the local doctor on the next day and he has given some tablets. I asked him the name of the tablet. He showed me the prescriptions, it was Bruben.

So I told the Paediatrician the bleeding is due to Bruben. induced haemorrhage and it can be treated conservatively. There was no bleeding after 48 hours of admission and the patient was discharged. After this incident I write some mild pain killer for the patients post operatively at the time of discharge.

24.1.2. PILES OPERATED POST OPERATIVE BLEEDING ON 3rd DAY.

I operated a lady assistant Professor in one of the city colleges in Dr.Fenn clinic. On the 3rd post operative day she passed motion and had severe bleeding per anus. Dr.Fenn called me to see the case. I went and saw the case there is blood leakage from the anus. I asked the patient what happened. She has said while washing after motion she palpated the threads and pulled out one of the three threads and had severe bleeding since then. Before my training in colorectal surgery, I used to leave the pedicles ligated catgut long which will be seen outside. Since 1982, I do not leave the thread and in my technique now the wound is sutured and there will be no raw area. I told Dr.Fenn the case to be taken to the theatre immediately. Dr.Fenn said the instruments have to be autoclaved and it will take at least 45 minutes. I told him I need one Proctoscope, two artery forceps, a needle holder and scissors which can be put in antiseptic solution for 10 minutes. In the mean time we will transfer the case to the theatre. I washed up changed the theatre dress for surgery. Under pudendal block, I passed the Proctoscope the bleeder from 3 o'clock pedicle was identified transfixed and ligated. The bleeding has stopped. Dr.Fenn appreciated the way in which I have managed the case with minimum instruments. In emergency situation like this we have to adopt a compromised attitude as far as the sterilization is concerned.

24.1.3. POST OPERATIVE BLEEDING ON THE DAY OF DISCHARGE.

A patient from Coimbatore area was operated for piles. He is a diabetics and hypertensive. After correction of these conditions he was operated. I did rectal examination on the 6th post operative day and told the patient that he can be discharged on his next day and he can go home in the evening. When I came for night rounds the dressing was found soaked with blood. When I asked nurse how long he has bleeding and who has changed the dressing. The hospital staff did not say anything. I examined the case, the bleeding is from the raw area only and not from the pedicles. I packed the area, went for night rounds came back and removed the pack after 45 minutes. The bleeding has stopped and advised the patient to lie down in the bed for the whole night. Now the nurse said that he has gone out with our operation theatre staffs for lunch by auto and came only after 3PM Since then the bleeding present. The patient said it is his fault by taking them by auto. They first refused to come but I only compelled them to come to hotel as a token of gratitude for the work they have done for me. I told him for the work we pay them. You need not give anything to them more. Anyhow you stay tomorrow also and go in the evening.

24.1.4. BIKE RIDING ON THE 8th POST OPERATIVE DAY.

A Doctor who has just finished Diploma in Anaesthesia came to me for piles. I examined it was a second degree piles which can be treated by rubber band ligation. But he said he is leaving for U.S.A. within a month and requested me to operate the piles. His parents are well known to me. I talked with them about the rubber band ligation and the need for second Ligation. They also said you operate and let him go to U.S.A after one month, so that we need not worry for the piles. I operated him and discharged after he passed motion on the 3rd post operative day. I asked him take complete bed rest and come for review after one week for rectal examination. He came to my clinic with a motor bike key. I asked him how he has come from his house. He said a friend came to see me and I dropped him in the central bus stand in the bike and I came here. I told him because you had a bike raiding and after rectal examination also you have to go home by bike, I am not doing rectal examination today. You come to vadamalayan hospital in the morning all 8.30 tomorrow in car; I will do the rectal examination. When I was in Vadamalayan hospital for night rounds, his mother rang up to Vadamalayan hospital and told me that her son immediately after return from your clinic went to toilet and he passed blood and fell down unconsciously. Now he is conscious and can we come to vadamalayan hospital now to see you. I asked her to come by car and I will be waiting for you. I saw the patient, he had bleeding from the raw area and the pedicle was normal. I admitted the patient, sedated him and started IV fluid, gave injection Vitamin k and Calcium gluconate. When I saw him in the morning at 6 AM he was comfortable and no bleeding.

I asked him to be in the hospital on that day and go home on his next day. If I have done rectal examination on that day in my clinic, they might have attributed the bleeding only because of rectal examination. Luckily I have not done the rectal examination. He saw me before leaving U.S.A.

24.1.5. CARDIAC ARREST DURING POST OPERATIVE RECTAL EXAMINATION.

A Lady Doctor, who was my house Surgeon, brought her father for piles treatment. He had 2nd degree piles which can be treated without surgical method. But the patient insisted that surgery should be done as he has come from Singapore for the treatment. So I did the surgery. On the 6th post operative day I did rectal examination in the room. The patient developed cardiac arrest. I asked the nurse to bring injection tray and gave adrenaline and cortisone injections, oxygen was given through mask and started I.V. fluid. The pulse rate gradually came to normal. By this time the patient's wife smelled that some problem to her husband and started crying, though her daughter was inside the room. I asked her to come to the room and showed her husband and said he is alright now. After this incident, I stopped doing rectal examination in the room. I do it in SOT where all resuscitation items are available.

24.1.6. PATIENT DEMONSTRATED THE BLEEDING TO EVERY BODY.

Rubber band ligation was done for second degree Piles. He wanted to stay 2 days in the hospital. Next day of Rubber Band ligation, he had bleeding per Rectum when he passed motion after my morning rounds.

He found out that straining at toilet results in bleeding. So he started demonstrating the bleeding to the people who had come to see him. The hospital nurse told him to lie down in the bed and don't strain. Still he was doing that, when I came for night rounds the duty nurse told me about what has happened in the day time. Now I told the patient that he needs to be in I.C.U. where no visitors are allowed and you cannot demonstrate the bleeding. As routine, drip was started and monitor was fixed in I.C.U. When I saw him in my morning rounds at 8.A.m. he said there was no bleeding after he came to I.C.U. and asked whether he would be transferred to his room. I said, yes I can, provided you promise me that you will not strain and demonstrate the bleeding to the visitors. He agreed and he was transferred to the room. After observation for one more day he was discharged.

24.1.7. DISTRIC EDUCATION OFFICER (D.E.O) WITH BLEEDING PILES.

One D.E.O was waiting to see me in my clinic. During that waiting period he went twice to the toilet. The way to toilet is through my consultation area. When he went for the 3rd time, the patient who was in my consultation room, was examined and waiting for discussion. I asked him to wait for some time, and told him that I will see that person who has gone for the toilet. When the D.E.O.came back from the toilet I asked him why he has gone to toilet for three times within this short period. He said he had a feeling of Defecation but when I went to the toilet only blood comes. While talking with me the blood was trickling down. So I asked him to lie on the examination table and I saw the bleeding is from prolapsing piles.

After examination, I told him he needs surgery for prolapsing piles at an earliest time. He said he has come prepared for surgery and ready to get admitted that day itself. I told him I can't do surgery tomorrow as I am going for conference to Hyderabad by 7.30 A.M. Flight from Madurai.

Even if I do surgery in early hours, my service will not be available for 3 days. If you get operated in vadamalayan hospital by some other surgeon, I will look after you after my return or you see some other doctor and get operated in their Hospital. He said I wanted to be under your care after surgery. So I ask another surgeon to operate in Vadamalayan hospital and after return from Hyderabad, I followed him post operatively and discharged him on the 6th post operative day. This patient had faith on me and wanted to be operated by me, but he cannot wait till I return due to bleeding, however I looked after him after my return from the conference and the follow up treatment was given by me. Later he referred 2 or 3 cases to me for piles treatment.

24.1.8. PILES WITH SEVERE ANAEMIA- ADMISSION AFTER 2 DAY.

A patient, astrologist, came to Vadamalayan hospital to see me at 8-30 am. I will usually be there, for patients who need sigmoidoscopy or some minor surgical procedures. I examined him; he had prolapsing piles with severe anaemia. Sigmoidoscopy was normal. I advised him admission for blood transfusion and Surgery. He said he will be coming after 2 days probably due to astrological factors. But I wrote admission in my O P. ticket. He had syncope attack while waiting for the settlement of bill for sigmoidoscopy. By that time I left Vadamalayan hospital. The duty doctor rang up to me and said the patient had syncope attack. I directed him to admit him Sedate him and start Blood.

When I came back at 2-30pm from G.R.H. the patient was in the waiting hall and my instructions were not carried over. When I asked the duty doctor why blood was not started, he said the patient was not willing for admission so the instructions were not carried over. I told him in that case you might have informed me or send the patient home why you allowed him to stay in the hospital from 9 am. For that duty doctor could not answer. Now I asked the patient to get admitted and have the treatment. Again the patient was particular to come after 2 days. I told him if you are not willing for admission now, you can go home and come back after 2 days. He came back after 2days, blood transfusion was given, operated and went home without any complication. Probably his astrological calculation for admission may be correct.

24.1.9. PILES WITH HAEMOGLOBIN 4G % OPERATED UNDER LOCAL.

One of my relatives from Tirunelveli came for piles treatment. He had prolapsing piles. His Hb was 4 G %'. Sigmoidoscopy was normal. I advised surgery but the anaesthetist said improve the Hb level by blood transfusion. As I have seen the bleeding from the prolapsing piles, there is no question of improving the Hb level with blood because it will take at least one week for Hb improvement by that time the bleeding may occur and Hb may come down.

So I did piles surgery under pudental nerve block and blood transfusion was given in the post operative period. He was discharged with advice of iron tablets and vitamins and asked him to come after 10 days for review. The level of Hb was 6 G%. Later he brought his wife for treatment of cancer breast.

24.1.10. PILES OPERATED- CONSUMERS FORUM.

A 58 years male patient was referred to me by the local general practitioner for bleeding per rectum. I examined the patient; it was a case of prolapsing piles. Sigmoidoscopy up to 25 cm was normal. I sent the patient to his doctor with all the findings with the advice for surgery. The patient was again referred to me for surgery. This is what routinely I do. When the patient required surgery, his doctor will decide to whom the patient to be sent for surgery. I did the necessary investigations and did surgery for piles. Next day of surgery he devolved retention of urine. So catheterization was done and kept one day for continuous urinary drain. When the catheter was removed on the 3rd post operative day, again he developed retention of urine. Urologist Dr.Varadarajen saw the case and advised Cystoscopy. After getting consent for Cystocopy, it was done by him under local. There was enlargement of median lobe of Prostate and he suggested surgery. The patient, his wife, and son had agreed for surgery. Prostatectomy was done by Dr.Varadarajan. There was excessive bleeding from the Prostatic bed. I was informed and I also joined the operating team. The Prosthetics bed was packed again and kept for 10 minutes and pack was removed. The bleeding stopped and the wound was closed. The patient was shifted from operation theatre and shown to the relatives and he was kept in I.C.U. for observation and the patient died after 8 hours of surgery.

The patient's three sons went to consumer's forum. Their allegation was, his father has come to me for only consultation but I admitted him and operated in the same day. A second operation was done on the 4th day (they mean Cystoscopy) and again after 3 days (Prostatectomy) and patient died on the operation table. But he was kept in lCU for one day and then only the death was declared. They also said all the three operations were done without their consent and demanded 5 Lacks compensation. I sent the copy of the case sheet, which clearly showed the patient was admitted on the second visit, operated for piles on the next day of admission after getting the consent from one of his sons in the case sheet. The Cystoscopy was done by Dr.Varadarajan the chief urologist in GRH. The 3nd time the patient was taken to operation theatre for Prostatectomy which was also done by Dr.Varadarajen. In all these occasions one of the patient's sons had signed the consent from. After Prostatectomy, the patient was seen by all the members of his family who were in the hospital at that time before the patient was taken to I.C.U. So surgery was not done on the same day of consultation. Piles surgery was done by me. Cystoscopy and Prostatectomy were done by the urologist. The patient was seen by all the members of the family available at that time, before the patient was sent to I.C.U. In all the three occasions the consent was signed by one of the patient's sons. Now that person also signed in this legal petition, and so I prayed this petition may be rejected. After going through the records the case was dismissed stating false allegation.

24.1.11. PILES OPERATED OUT SIDE – FAECAL INCONTINENCE.

A patient was brought to my clinic by taxi and the relatives said the patient cannot be shifted to the consultation room as there is faecal soiling in his body. This was the only occasion I came out of my Consultation room to the road and saw the patient.

I suspected faecal incontinence. When asked the patient how it had occurred he said he was operated for piles at Virudunagar. Since then he cannot control the faces. He was admitted in Vadamalayan hospital. I examined him the external anal orifice was patulous and there was evidence of damage to the internal anal sphincter. I told the patient that he needs three operations colostomy, sphincter repair, and colostomy closure, and the total treatment time will be around four months. After colostomy you can go home and come for sphincter repair and then for colostomy closure. He agreed for operation. So I did colostomy under local and the faecal soiling was completely controlled and he was discharged with an advice to come after 10 days for assessing whether the infection has controlled or the antibiotics to be changed. After six weeks sphincter repair was done and the patient was discharged with the advice is come for colostomy closure. The colostomy was closed after 3 weeks He was in the hospital for some time to make sure that the sphincters are functioning well and no faecal soiling. I asked the patient, how he was so prompt in coming for review on the dates fixed, from Virudunagar.

He said, sir, you have already explained about three surgeries and the total time for treatment may be around four months. So I sold my house at Virudunagar and stayed in the next street of your house with my wife. I used that money for lending to known persons and we lived here with that money. I appreciated the way by which he got the money for the treatment with a determined mind to have treatment for incontinence, instead of borrowing money, and he was lending money to other people and the capital amount was saved.

24.2. FISTULA IN ANO.

24.2.1. VETERINARY DOCTOR - POST OPERATIVE BLEEDING.

A veterinary doctor was operated by Dr.C.K. He had bleeding from the wound in the evening. Dr. C.K asked me to see the case during my night rounds. I went a little earlier for the night rounds and saw the patient who was in special ward; the dressing was completely soaked with blood. I immediately transferred him to emergency theatre and removed the dressing. When the blood colt was removed from the wound, an active arterial bleeding from the edge of the wound was detected which was ligated under local. He came for review for three or four times till the wound has healed well.

24.2.2. A PATIENT DEMANDED MEDICAL FITNESS CERTIFICATE.

A person working in the Co-operative department came for consultation for Fistula. I examined him, investigated and told him he needs surgery for the fistula and may need one month rest. He said he is on leave for his daughter's marriage and I have applied for extension of leave and in that period I will get operated for fistula. I told him it is better to join duty now and come for surgery after one or two months later as it is not an emergency. If you extend the leave there is every possibility that you may be transferred. He insisted that surgery to be done now itself and so I did the surgery. At the expiry of the previous leave, I recommend one month leave. Now his place was filled by some other person as he had extended his leave. As the wound has not healed, he wanted one more month medical leave and recommended the medical leave for one month. One week after submitting the second medical leave application with my medical certificate, he came to my clinic and asked medical fitness certificate. He said the higher authority agreed to post him in a vacant place and asked him to get the medical fitness certificate. I asked him to bring the previous medical leave certificate and I will give the fitness certificate. He said that is with the higher official office and I cannot get it. I told him that I have recommended one month leave but within one week you wanted the fitness certificate which I cannot give. He got angry by my statement and said you are talking like a perfect man to me, you know that I am a Gazetted officer. I told him yes I am a perfect man in all aspect and I am a Gazetted office from the day one when I joined duty in Government service. You might have got this rank after working for more than twenty years or so. I will not give fitness unless you bring the old leave certificate. After some arguments, he said I will complaint to D.M.S. and see that you are transferred from Madurai. I told him that I am working under D.M.E. and you have to give complaint to D.M.E. and not to D.M.S. You can report anybody that I refused to give fitness certificate, and now you leave the place as I have to see the patients who are waiting. Sometimes we have to face such situations. Knowing the rules, I told him first to join duty after his daughter's marriage and after one or two months have surgery for fistula. Still I do not know why he was particular about to have surgery at that period, and had leave extended.

24.2.3. PATIENT DID NOT WANT SURGERY AT VADAMALAYAN HOSPITAL.

A lady patient working in a departmental store had fistula and after examination I advised surgery for fistula. She agreed for surgery and asked me where I will be doing surgery. I said at Vadamalayan hospital. She said she did not want surgery at Vadamalayan hospital because her husband died there due to heart attack. If I am admitted there I will be thinking about my husband's suffering. I agreed with her sentiment and told her in that case I could operate in one hospital at Anna Nagar which is nearer to your house. She said she is alone and no child. The patient was admitted and surgery was fixed on the next day. One person came to my clinic and asked me what disease that lady is having and what surgery I am going to do. Since I knew that lady is a widow having no child, I asked him who is he and what is his relation to that patient He said he is known to her, immediately I asked him to get out from my clinic as he is not willing to reveal who is he and said that he is known to her. I told him if you are not willing to reveal who you are, why should I reveal the medical condition of my patient and reveal the professional secrecy to others without the permission from the patient. Next day after the surgery, I told her that one person came to my clinic yesterday and asked about your disease and the nature of operation. She said I had not told anything to anybody about my surgery. We have to be careful to any person coming without the patient and ask about the nature of the disease.

24.3. FISSURE IN ANO IN A PATIENT OF 120 K.G. WEIGHT.

A patient from Aranthangi came for the treatment of chronic fissure in ano. He was posted for anal dilatation and excision of hypertrophied anal papilla and skin tag under general anaesthesia at 6 AM on the next day. The patient was brought to the operation theatre by a stretcher and I asked him to move to the operation table. While moving to the operation table, he adjusted himself with pressure by both hands on the operation table and the operation table has given away and broken across in the centre. Fortunately myself and the theatre assistant hold him and prevented him from falling down and the patient was transferred to stretcher. The patient was stable and he is more concerned about the damage of operation table because of his weight. I told him don't bother about that. Do you want the surgery to be done today or want to be postponed. He said I have come from Aranthangi and my relations have come and I cannot come on some other day so if possible operate today itself. I asked the anaesthetist whether he is willing to give anaesthesia, he said we have done many cases in the stretcher and so there is no problem in this case. Anal dilation, excision of skin tag and hypertrophied anal papilla were done under G.A. in the stretcher.

24.4. PERIANAL ABSCESS.

24.4.1. LOCAL ANAESTHETIC REACTION.

My Barber's son in law had perianal abscess and decided to do incision and drainage under local anaesthesia. As the routine skin test for lignocaine were done 30 minutes before surgery. There was no evidence of skin reaction to lignocaine. So field block was done with lignocaine. Suddenly the patient had developed air hunger and restlessness and allergic rashes in the skin. Immediately injection Adrenaline and Decadron were given. Nasal oxygen was started.

The patient's father in law (my Barber) was called inside and told him what has happened and now he is recovering. If he completely recovers within half an hour I will do I & D., otherwise we will do under general anaesthesia after wards. The patient completely recovered from allergic reaction and I & D was done after 45 minutes. I told the patient and the Barber that he should not be given lignocaine injection in his life time.

24.4.2. PERIANAL ABSCESS JUST FOUR DAYS BEFORE MARRIAGE.

A girl was brought to me with pain in the anal region and fever of 4 days duration. She was treated by the local doctor without examine her. When the pain was unbearable she was brought to me by her mother. I examined her and advised incision and drainage immediately, and if necessary surgery for fistula some time later. The patient's mother said her marriage function is fixed within next four days. I told them in that cases incision and drainage itself may cure the condition and in some cases a fistula may develop later for which surgery is needed. So I told them now I will do incision and drainage, let her have marriage and after 2 or 3 months if necessary surgery can be done. After marriage, the couple came to my clinic. On examination, the fistula has developed. I explained the condition to the couple. They were quite understandable and agreed for surgery. They came after one month for fistula surgery.

24.4.3. BLEEDING AFTER INCISION AND DRAINAGE.

A building contractor, living near my house came with perianal abscess. He is diabetic and so I told him to get admitted in Vadamalayan hospital and get the investigations done before I come for the morning rounds and I will do incision and drainage under local. He agreed to stay in the hospital and have all the investigations. I did incision and drainage under local.

When I came for night rounds the nurse said she changed the dressing three times because of blood stained discharge. I examined him in S.O.T. There was active bleeding from the cut end of a vessel which was ligated. I asked the nurse why she has not informed me, the patient said I only requested them not to inform you and told her let him see me when he comes for night rounds. The patient becomes alright and fistula has not devolved in this case.

25. COLONIC PATHOLOGY.

25.1. MULTIPLE POLYPOSIS COLI.

A schedule trip girl of 12 years came for bleeding per rectum and anaemia. Sigmoidoscopy revealed multiple polyposis. Colonoscopy showed Polyps up to ascending colon. The patient was prepared for subtotal colectomy with ileorectal anastomosis. Her Hb was brought to 6 G % with supportive therapy and one unit of blood. The anaesthetist, Dr. Nirmaladevi, was quite reluctant to give anaesthesia for such a major surgery. I told her 3 units of blood are ready for surgery and in the immediate post operative period. If I give the blood preoperatively, I am sure that the Hb level will not increase, because she is bleeding. Somehow the anaesthetist was convinced and gave anaesthesia. Subtotal colectomy with ileorectal anastomosis was done as the rectum was free from polyps. Even the polyps occur in the rectum, can be easily seen by proctoscopy or sigmoidoscopy.

Post operatively faecal fistula occurred and was treated conservatively. I told the mother to bring her for periodical review for rectal polyps. She came after 2 years with her parents. I did proctoscopy and Sigmoidoscopy and the rectum was free from polyps. I took this opportunity to examine her parents with sigmoidoscopy and they were found normal. They told me that they have come to see me to ask whether she can marry. Even if I say no, I am sure that she will be married and so I said yes for the marriage.

25.2. ACUTE ULCERATIVE COLITIS.

A worker in local Tamil news paper was admitted in GRH for acute stage of Ulcerative Colitis. There was no attendant for him. He was put on D.I.L. (Dangerously ill list) and informed the relatives to the address given at the time admission. After 4 or 5 days one person came and left within 3 days. We treated the patient without any relatives with him. Fortunately there was marked improvement in his condition. The acute stage was managed effectively and after two months I told the patient that he needs treatment with tablets which will be available in outpatient. He said he will go after one week. I discharged him after one week without anybody with him. For this disease we can give tablets for 15 days in one prescription.

He came for 2 or 3 months and then he has not come for review. When I was going by bus to Chennai, the bus stopped at Samayapram near Trichy. One person came to me and said his name is Anandan and he was treated by me in GRH about out 5 years back. I could not recognize him. Then he said he was a worker in Tamil news paper. Now I was able to identify him and asked him how is his health He said he is continuing the tablets and the dosage were markedly reduced, talking one table twice a week. He said he has completed law and now working under a senior lawyer and going to Chennai regarding a case in high court. I was happy to see him as a professional man with a good healthy body. I just recollected how seriously he was admitted in the hospital without any attending person and kept him in the hospital for more than two months.

25.3. ULCERATIVE COLITIS NOT RESPONDING TO MEDICAL TREATMENT.

Mrs. Lakshmi Devi from Dindugal came to my clinic for the treatment of acute attack of passing blood and mucus per rectum. Sigmoidoscopy showed acute inflammation even beyond 25cms from anus, and I took biopsy. The report came as Acute Phase of Ulcerative colitis. She was treated by medical treatment for three months, but there was no satisfactory improvement in the symptoms, and her general condition was going down. She developed anaemia and hypoprotinemia. She was admitted and had supportive treatment with Human Albumin, IV amino acids. Vitamins and iron were given IV. I told her husband about her condition and need for total Coloproctectomy and ileostomy. I explained the need for surgery to the patient also. She is an educated lady and understands the need for the surgery and agreed for ileostomy.

Total Coloproctectomy and ileostomy was done with four units of blood during surgery. The post operative period was uneventful. The ileostomy Bag was fixed on the table itself and we tought her how to manage Ileostomy bag. When she came for review, I asked, was there any reason for that acute episode of ulcerative colitis. She said she saw one of her close relation got fire accident in the kitchen and died. Now I understand that

Psychological trauma was the cause for the acute episode of the disease. During ASICO 99 in Madurai, Colorectal workshop was conducted in Vadamalayan hospital. At that time she was shown for ileostomy to the delegates and there was a video discussion all about the management of ileostomy. This patient answered all the questions asked by the delegates in English. I was very happy to see and hear my patient is talking with the delegates in English. To be happy in life, you must be happy with your work and that is the only way in our medical profession.

25.4. TOTAL PROCTOCOLECTOMY WITH ILEOSTOMY. MARITAL PROBLEMS.

A patient from Madurai had acute phase of Ulcerative colitis. I discussed with the patient and his wife about the nature of the disease and said we will give medical treatment for 2-3 months and if there is no improvement, then surgery has to be done. They were living in a joined family. On hearing the duration of treatment and may need a major operation, all three brothers of this patient decided to have partition of the property, that leads to mental strain to the patient and acute episode persists even with high dose drugs. The patient himself demanded surgery. I explained the nature of surgery and the need for ileostomy. The patient and his wife agreed for surgery and total Proctocolectomy and Ileostomy was done. He was completely cured from the disease. After one year he had a confidential discussion with me about the marital relationship and sex with his wife. I asked him to come with his wife in the next visit. Both of them had counselling when they came for review. During discussion she said that sometimes faecal soiling occurs during sex and that is very embracing for me and so I avoided sex. I talked with them about the different positions of sexual activity and such embracing situations can be prevented. They came after two years with a male child and they said they live happily in all aspects.

25.5. PELVIC COLON GROWTH.

A bank employee, widow, was referred to me for the management of Pelvic colon growth. She was brought to me by her co-workers in the Bank. I was happy to see them and they said her husband died and no child, so we have to help her. I told them that she needs surgery. One of them asked me what will be the approximate amount. I told them the approximate amount including the room rent. The operation went on smoothly and the post operative period was uneventful. After suture removal I told her you can go on the next day. When I came in the afternoon for surgery for some other case, the nurse told me that the attenders said that they don't have enough money now and pay the balance when they come for review. I told the nurse no problem, you collect the amount they give and give them the receipt for that and the balance amount write in the discharge summery case sheet and also tell me the amount due. This sometimes happens because I tell then only approximate amount and sometimes unexpectedly the amount may go higher. In these situations, I tell the hospital staff to collect the hospital charges and for my charge get whatever they give and the balance amount you write in the discharge summary case sheet and tell patient also about the balance amount, so that the patient can bring at the time of review. In such cases, when they enter my consultation room, they place the balance amount due on the table. This bank employee came for review, I examined her, gave some instructions. But she has not given the balance amount. I told her she has to pay the balance amount which was due at time of discharge. She told me that the person, who stayed in the hospital, told her that all the bills were settled. I showed her the balance mount written in the discharge summary case sheet. She told me that she had pledged her gold chain in the bank and gave all the money to him. I asked her how much amount she has given. She said double the amount of total expenditure in the hospital. I said the total amount would have been much less the amount you have given to him. Even then he told the reception counter that he has not enough money. I told the nurse in the reception; now give them the receipt for the amount received and the balance amount you write in the discharge summary case sheet. I showed her the amount due. She said she has no money and will bring the money when she comes for next time. I told her total expenditure for the treatment and amount paid and the balance amount. When she came for second review she paid the balance. Now out of curiosity I asked her what that person said. She said I have checked the total expenditure and the amount paid and the balance amount and asked him about the rest of the money. He agreed to give the money from the next month's pay. After this incidence, I told the nurse in vadamalayan hospital, you tell the amount due to the patient and some body may pay it. Now the patient will know how much they have paid. In this case, my patient did not know that nobody will help anybody without monitory benefits, is the trend now.

26. RECTAL CONDITIONS.

26.1. REPEATED PREOPERATIVE BIOPSIES WERE NON MALIGANENT.

Mr. Joseph Viswasam, a co-operative Society employee, came to colorectal outpatient for bleeding per Rectum. He had proliferative growth at 8cm from the anal verge, biopsy was taken. The report was non malignant. The Biopsy was repeated and the specimen was sent to Madurai Medical College Pathology department and to the Private Biopsy centre. This time also both reports are non malignant. Though I suspected malignancy in this case, the three reports were non malignant. So I discussed with him and his family members about the possibility of malignancy and told them now I will do excision the whole mass and sent for biopsy for different places. If the report comes as malignancy, he should undergo abdominoperineal resection and permanent Colostomy. The patient agreed. Excision biopsy was done under anaesthesia. I sent the specimen to Dr. RadhaKrishnan at Thanjavure also. From all the 3 places the report came as malignant. Now I told the patient about the report of cancer and advised surgery. He agreed and had abdominoperineal Resection (APR) and pelvic Colostomy. He had some urinary bladder complaints for that I referred him to urologist for further management.

26.2. A P RESECTION FOR 10TH STANDARD GIRL.

A 15 years girl came for bleeding per rectum. She had an ulcer in the rectum at 7 cm from anal verge. Biopsy was done and the report was Adeno carcinoma Rectum. She was a 10th standard student in corporation school. After explaining the nature of surgery, I did Abdominoperineal resection and pelvic colostomy. I advised her to wear colostomy bag which I got as samples from the company, when I was attending the conference. After some time I was told that she was not wearing the colostomy bags. When I asked about this, she said she knows when the colostomy was about to act and she immediately left to toilet to clean. The school teachers had permitted her at any time to leave the class room without asking.

Every time she wants admission I admitted her. Like that she was admitted for some wake complaints one year after the surgery. I saw her in the ward on the day of admission and next day. The 2nd day of her admission was my operation day; I have not gone to the female ward in the night as no female patient was operated on that day. Next day before going to Colorectal OP I went to female ward to see her. She asked me why I have not seen her in the previous day.

I told her yesterday was operation day and the list was heavy so I have not come to see you. She said whatever may be, you must have come to see me. As she was speaking to me her pulse became weak and I asked the nurse to start the IV drip and gave other instructions. Now I know that she is dying. So I left the place and went to Colorectal OP and asked the house surgeon to be in the ward to see the girl Rani, within 10 minutes the house surgeon said that she died. Though her name was Rani, she is a Muslim girl.

Dear Rani I can say the only following statement why I didn't see you on my operation day: I might have skipped attending to you to attend someone else. But that is not because I was ignoring you. It was only must because I felt someone else needed a quicker intervention than you.

Surprisingly, cancer rectum occurs in young female of Muslims. The reason for that is to be found out. Once Dr.Parasuraman, Professor of surgery in Coimbatore Medical College, took me for ward rounds said he had a case of cancer rectum in a teen age girl. I asked him is it Muslim girl. He was surprised to hear that question and said yes, and asked me have you seen cancer rectum in such a young girl. I said I have seen 3 cases in teenage girls and all of them were Muslim and unfortunately the prognosis is poor.

26.3. A P RESECTION IN A LOADED RECTUM.

Those days before the peglec has come to the market preoperative bowel preparation was a tedious procedure. Fluid diet for 3 days, tape water enema twice a day and in the morning of the day of surgery so totally 5 enemas will be given so that there should be no faecal material in the large intestine. In addition oral antibiotics and Metronidozol were given for 3 days. One patient had bowel preparation for AP resection. When the abdomen was opened the colon was found loaded with faecal mass. I had half a mind to close the abdomen. It was at that period papers were published whether the bowel preparation is necessary for colorectal surgery and so I thought I can do surgery for that case. Unfortunately the patient died in the 2nd post operative day. When death occurred like this we discuss whether it is a preventable death. When we are discussing with the assistant, PG and CRRI in the ward, one patient said on the previous day of surgery, the patient's relatives gave briyani and chicken to the patient. I told him not to eat, as tomorrow you have surgery. The patient's relatives told that after surgery they will not allow food for 3 or 4 days so let him take now. I asked him why he had not told me when I came for night rounds. He said that you may scold the patient and after that the patient will squarrel with me and so I kept silent. I told him if you had said that I would have cancelled the surgery, and now see he died. This patient is a poor man coming from a remote village, uneducated people, cannot understand why we say starvation before surgery.

26.4. HAD TWO CHILDREN AFTER AP RESECTION.

Mr.Logosundaram unmarried man was operated for carcinoma of rectum. He had 5 FU injection post operatively. After 5 years he asked me whether he can marry I said, as you had completed five years after surgery so can marry, provided your penile erection function is normal.

He said that is alright. The marriage function was conducted at Meenakshi Amman temple at about 10.30AM. The wedded couple directly came to my clinic at 11.30 AM for blessing. I blessed the couple and told the bride if you have any doubt about health conditions of your husband you can contact me. She said the bride groom has told her about the surgery even before the marriage was fixed. Mr.Logasundaram came to GRH with sweet packet in his hand. I asked him, the child is Male or female.

He was surprised and asked me how you know. I told him the happiness in your face and the sweet packet in your hand I guessed that you became a father. He distributed the sweet to all the members in colorectal clinic. After 2 years he came back and I asked whether he had another child. He said yes delivered yesterday. I told him to bring up more than two children will be more difficult and so come after 6 months when the baby had grown well for vasectomy. He came after 6 months; I did the vasectomy for him. Vasectomy for birth control in a cancer patient, particularly after AP Resection, done 10 years back is a rare occasion. Probably I was the only surgeon who had such an opportunity.

26.5. AP RESECTION FOR A YOUNG MAN.

I operated a unmarried Muslim man for cancer rectum and he had injection 5 FU full course. He got a job at Chennai and every year he was coming at 8.30 AM to Vadamalayan hospital for review and returned on the same day. At one visit he asked me whether he can marry. I said after 5 years from the time of surgery. After 2 years I got a reply post card from his father whether his son can get married now. The name of the father given in the letter was different from the name of the patient's father which I remembered at that time. I wrote in the reply card that this cannot be revealed in the letter, you come in person. When the patient came for review I told him about the letter sent by your father. He said that is not his father's name probably somebody would have written to know about my health.

After 5 years of surgery, when he came for the review, he asked whether he can marry now. I saw the record he had completed 5 years and there was no evidence of recurrence so I said yes you can. The marriage was fixed at Aeral.

I told him in the same day I am coming to Tirunelveli to attend a marriage, from there I will be coming to just to see you as a bride groom. But my driver came only at 9 AM even though I asked him to come at 6AM. So I not attended both marriages and stopped the driver from the work.

26.6. GOVT. DOCTORS ARE NOT DOING WORK. REMARK FROM A PRIVATE SURGEON.

A patient was referred from Dindugal to Colorectal op in G.R.H. I examined the patient and did Biopsy and the diagnosis of cancer rectum was confirmed. I discussed with the patient and his wife about the nature of the disease and the need for surgery and also about the colostomy. They agreed and I did abdominoperineal Resection with colostomy. Trial catheter removal was done on the 7th post operative day. The patient could not pass urine so the catheter was reintroduced. Usually I remove the perineal sutures when the patient comes for the review after 8 days. So the patient was discharged with the catheter and perineal sutures. I asked the patient to come after 8 days for the removal of perineal sutures and the Bladder catheter. This patient went to see his doctor at Dindugal. That doctor saw the catheter and the perineal suture and told the patient that the doctors in Government service are irresponsible; see that you were discharged with catheter and perineal sutures.

He removed the catheter and perineal sutures. This patient was readmitted in medical side with retention of urine and convulsion from casualty. Medical side peoples sent the patient to colorectal ward. The Bladder was markedly distended and the perineal wound had given way. The blood urea and the serum creatinine were very high I asked the urologist, Dr.Varadarajen to see the case. The patient was put on continuous Bladder drainage and treated as advised by the urologist. After recovery from uraemia the perineal wound was sutured.

After the patient the patient becomes alright I asked the patient who removed the catheter and perineal sutures. He said the Dindugal doctor on the next day of discharge from here; I saw him and he removed the catheter and the sutures. Then I went 2 or 3 times for continuous tripling of urine. The doctor said it will be alright within a week without examining him. I asked the patient to see the Dindugal doctor and tell him that Govt. doctors are more responsible in treating the patients and they know when to remove the catheter and when to remove the perineal sutures. I don't know whether he met the doctor afterwards.

When he came for review once he said personally that he used to take non vegetarian food daily but now my wife is not giving non vegetarian food, please tell her about that. After some time I call her and said the patient needs nutritional food particularly eggs, mutton and chicken (at that time the chicken was costlier). She said I am giving two eggs in a week, once a week mutton and sometimes chicken. I have two children I have to give food for them also. I have limited income with that I am managing. The surgeons are very proud of saying that they have done so many major complicated cases and they forget the socioeconomic impact on the family following the successful surgery.

26.7. PARASTOMAL HERNIA REPAIR AFTER 13 YEARS OF APR.

Mrs. Arundathi was operated in Dr.KAS Hospital for cancer rectum 13 years back. She was an active member of Ostomates India Madurai branch. She had parastomal hernia and she wanted me to do surgery at Vadamalayan hospital. The reason for surgery was she couldn't fix the colostomy appliance properly and leakage of motion. It is a common condition after stoma but usually small and asked them to use a little larger size facet appliance I have not seen such a large size parastomal hernia. I informed Dr.KAS, my teacher about this case and she wanted me to operate in Vadamalayan hospital. He said she used to come for review, I thought of calling you to see her. Now she has come to you and you do the operation. I operated her and mesh was used for the repair.

26.8. APR DONE. THE PATIENT WAS FORCED TO JOIN DUTY.

A patient from Keelakarai was operated for cancer rectum AP Resection and colostomy was done. He was working in a Govt.office in his place. I recommended medical leave for two months. For cancer patients we can recommend leave for six months. But the patient was otherwise normal except colostomy which is unavoidable for this condition. He thought that the co worker may feel uneasy to see him with colostomy. I told him after three months I will advise irrigation technique then you need colostomy appliance for safety purpose only. He was very particular not join duty. I told him you join duty and if you are not happy with your co-workers in the office I will recommend leave for three months and you do not assume that your colleagues will not accept you. With half minded he accepted my advice and got the fitness certificate and joined the duty. He came after 3 months for review, I asked him how you feel in the in the office after you joined duty. He said all people in the office are more affectionate with me and I am very happy to go to office. After six months he said he is very happy in the office and on office leave days I am little disturbed because I think how to spend the time in the house. When he retired from service asked me whether he can join a job in Tirunelveli. I said you must do some work after retirement, and then only you have an active life. He joined the job at Tirunelveli.

In this instance I could recollect that one doctor had hemiplegic attack and difficulty with speak. He was on physiotherapy for 3 months. He came to medical board for extension of leave. I was in the medical board as a member. He asked extension of leave for two months. He was my wife classmate. I told him if we recommend leave, you will be alone in the house as your children will go to school and your wife will be doing house works. If you join duty you can try to talk with the people in the department which itself is physiotherapy. You work in non clinical department and if you are not happy you come to the board we will recommend leave. He joined duty in Biochemistry department and posted as medical officer in G.R.H Biochemistry department. I saw him in the department he was much involved in the duty, his speech was much improved, and he thanked me for the advice given in the medical board.

26.9. PLANED APR. NO LESION AT OPERATION.

A tailor from nearby Srivalliputhur area was referred to colorectal op for the treatment of cancer rectum by the local doctor with the Biopsy report. I examined the patient he had an ulcerative lesion in the rectum about 6 CM from the anal verge. He was investigated and decided surgery. I discussed about the nature of surgery and colostomy. He agreed and posted for surgery. But due to some reason we not able to do surgery and posted for surgery in the next week. Totally 3 weeks has gone before I did surgery. After the abdomen was opened, assessment of local extension of the lesion and spread to the lymph nodes were done. I could not palpate the lesion from above and the pelvic aspect of rectum was normal. I asked the assistant to do rectal examination he said no growth was palpable. So I did the rectal examination no lesion was palpable. The lesion which I palpated in the OP was completely subsided. I did sigmoidoscopy in the operation table which was normal.

Normally I do rectal examination for all the cases on the previous day of surgery. In this particular case I have not done rectal examination on the previous day. The abdomen was closed without proceeding further. As the surgery was done under epidural anaesthesia I told the patient that colostomy was not done and I will talk to you in the ward. After the theatre was over I used to see the operated cases in the ward and give instructions to the ward nurse. After the ward works, I talked with the patient and told him I have not done the surgery because I couldn't make out the lesion during surgery. I will examine you every month for at least six months. As there was no lesion made out during six months follow up, I asked the patient to come to the hospital when bleeding occurs. I discussed with one of the responsible men in Grace Kennet hospital about the Biopsy report which was given by their Pathologist as adenocarcinoma. He said if you have the Biopsy report with you, give it to me. I will check the report with the pathologist. When I asked him after some time whether the pathologist reviewed the slid, he said he misplaced the report and it could not be traced. Even big people say lies to protect their pathologist.

26.10. AP RESECTION DONE PATHOLOGIST MISSED THE DIAGNOSIS.

A lady patient came to the colorectal OP for the treatment of cancer rectum. Biopsy was done in Christian medical college Vellore but the patient had come to Madurai for surgery. I did abdominoperineal resection and sent the excised specimen for Biopsy. The report was nonspecific ulcer no evidence of malignancy. I was a little upset. I went to the pathology department and discussed with them. They were very definite about their report. I saw our Biopsy registers there was no entry of previous Biopsy report, then I recollected that the patient had come with Biopsy from Vellore and that fact was already entered in case sheet with Biopsy number. I showed the case sheet to the pathologist. As I have sent the whole specimen, they did multiple sections. Still they said it is non malignant. The patient was discharged with a guilty mind and asked her to come for review every month for 6 months. After 6 months when she came there was a nodule in the perineal scar. I did excision Biopsy and now the report came as secondary deposit. Though I was happy to see the report as secondary deposit, as for the patient is concerned it is a bad prognostic point. Now I went to Pathology department and said this specimen was from the patient's perineal scar for which you had reported non malignant lesions from the whole specimen of AP resection. You have missed the lesion from the whole rectum but you have made out from a small nodule. Previously I was much worried that people may think that I am doing AP Resection for non malignant lesions to increase the number of APR. Now I have proven that I have done for cancer only.

I had a principle that blood for the elective surgery must be donated by the relatives of the patient. For this patient also one of her sons donated blood. I asked her what she had done for that son who had donated blood. She said I have given one buffalo which is giving 4 litres of milk every day. I saw her about 3 years after local excision of the perineal deposit. So I presume that in the scar is due to spill over of malignant cell during surgery.

26.11. THANKS GIVEING PARTY FOR COMPLETING 100 CASES OF APR.

I started colorectal department in 1982 December with one Paediatric Proctoscope and gradually the department was improved. There were 20 Proctoscopes,Sigmoidoscope, colonoscope, diagnostic laparoscope, Piles injection syringe, Rubber Band ligator,Cryo apparatus, Stapler gun for colon anatomises. The number of patient increased from 1 or 2 cases to 40 cases per one op day. The OP was conducted 3 days a week. Many people helped for the improvement of the department. I thank the Deans at that time, Deputy Superintendent Dr.A. Subramanian, Prof.and HOD. of surgery Dr.C.Raman, Prof and HOD. Of anaesthesia Dr.Viswanathan. I also thank the assistants in anaesthesia department, and all the Doctors and nurses who have worked in colorectal unit, theatre nurses and theatre assistants who have helped for the development of colorectal department. When I have Completed 100 cases of Abdominoperineal Resection without mortality, I took it as an opportunity to say thanks to them, and arranged a Thanks giving lunch at IMA hall on 24th December 1992. I invited them by saying just you come at your convenient time for lunch at IMA Hall on 24th December between 12.30 PM to 4 PM for the Thanks giving Lunch. The response was very good.

26.12. RECTO URETHRAL FISTULA.

A patient had Trans Vasical Prostatectomy in E.S.I. hospital Madurai. The patient developed recto urethral fistula. He was referred to colorectal op. The patient told me that the E.S.I. Doctor said one doctor has come from UK trained in G.R.H. but he also may not be able to treat you, anyhow I refer you see him. I took it as a challenge and started the treatment. I did colostomy to prevent contamination of urinary tract with faecal material. A Foleys catheter was passed for continuous Bladder drainage and kept in place for 3 weeks. The catheter was removed after 3 weeks. The patient had some problems for micturation because the Bladder was on continuous drainage and the Bladder tone regained slowly and dripping of urine was stopped. A micturating cysto urethrogram was done. It was normal and there was no urethral fistula or stricture. Barium enema was done through the non functioning lumen of the colostomy. There was no evidence of any fistula. The colostomy was closed and the patient was discharged after suture removal. I asked the patient to see the ESI hospital surgeon and show the discharge Summary and tell him that you were alright now, because the medical leave has to be recommended by him.

26.13. RECTO VAGINAL FISTULA.

A girl of about 18 years was brought by her mother for consultation regarding passing motion through the vagina. I examined the patient, she had congenital low Anorectal anomaly, Vestibular Anus. The anal sphincter control was normal. Her menstrual cycle was normal.

Abdominal Scan and CT abdomen were done to find out any other congenital abnormalities, and they were normal. I explained the condition to them and it is only a congenital anomaly which can be corrected. They agreed for correction and I did anal transposition. After 2 years the mother came to me and asked whether her daughter can be married now. I said yes, but if she becomes pregnant, tell the doctor that she had anal transposition for congenital anomaly so that they can avoid episiotomy and if there is any problem in delivery they can procedure with LSCS Without any delay. She got married and had normal delivery which was conducted by my wife. I gave the warning because if episiotomy was done there is every possibility of anal sphincter damage because the distance between the anus and the posterior aspect of vagina is narrow. If perineal tear occurs the same complication will occur. So the obstetrician has to balance between the normal delivery and LSCS.

27. OTHER RARE CONDITIONS.

27.1. EMERGENCY PNUMONECTOMY.

A patient from my native place had pulmonary lobectomy right side for pulmonary tuberculosis with haemoptysis, I was doing PG in 1969 at GRH at the time. He had recurrent severe Haemoptysis in1975 and decided emergency pnemonectomy on the same side by the thoracic surgeon Dr.V.Srinivason. The patient was admitted in Vadamalayan hospital and emergency Pnumonectomy was done. The patient needed 5 units of blood which were brought from private blood Bank. The patient was well to do person and his only daughter was married to a person working in Labour department.

The patient's wife, daughter, and son in law were present during surgery. Once the patient was shifted from the theatre, the son in law said he has to go for the duty at Trichy and come in the night. I was surprised to hear that and told him that we have to give money to the anaesthetist, blood bank and operation theatre charges and replace the drugs used in the theatre now. The surgeon and the assistant Bills can be settled later. He said he has no money now. I told him the surgery went on for more than two hours, by the time you might have made arrangements for the money. As the patient was from my place and my relative I can look after him but he has to pay the money. Normally only after the money was paid blood will be given from the blood Bank. In this case because I talked with them they have given the blood without payment. He said he will come within half an hour with money. As promised he came with money and settled that day account. It seems, because I know to them they might have thought that, the account can be settled at the time of discharge. The lesson I learned from this case, was even the case is a relation it is better to tell them certain amounts to be paid to the hospital on the day of surgery.

27.2. A CASE OF TUBEROSCLEROSIS.

One PG student got permission to go to library to get some references. On his way through the casualty he saw a case and out of curiosity he examined the case and found out bilateral renal mass. He asked me whether he can admit case in our unit as it is an interesting case. I said you request the casualty medical officer to admit in our unit as our old case. When the patient came to the ward I examined him. He was a low IQ man with multiple Sebaceous tumours in the face and bilateral cystic renal mass probably Polycystic kidney.

I referred to skin OP, they diagnosed as Tuberosclerosis and they suggested Neurological examination as the patient may have lesions in the spinal canal. I referred the patient to Neuro physician for neurological evaluation. They have written transfer the case to Neuro ward for neurological evaluation.

The patient was from Palani. Because of clinical interest, he was given a bed when he was transferred to Neuro ward he was asked to lie on the floor and bed was not given. He came back to our ward next day evening. The nurse told him you have to be there for some tests and after that they will send you back to this ward. He told the nurse I will be in this ward only other wise I will go back to Palani. The nurse asked him to come in the morning, the doctor may transfer you to this ward. This patient left the hospital in the evening itself and we did not know where he had gone. The patients who have clinical interesting conditions will not stay in the hospital if they have no problems.

27.3. HIND QUARTER AMPUTATION FOR GIANT CHONDROMA OF PELVIC BONE.

Mr. Muthuvel was admitted in ortho ward Dr.Devadoss unit in GRH for giant chondroma of pelvic bone. He had chronic constipation with loaded rectum, pelvic colon, descending colon and transverse colon. I discussed with Dr.Devadoss about diversion colostomy to avoid faecal contamination during surgery. Dr.Devadoss asked me to come to the theatre on the day of Hindquarter Amputation. Urologist Dr.Ravindranath also was present. During surgery the Bladder was opened and it was closed by the Urologist. A small rectal tear was closed by me. Since preoperative colostomy was done there was no faecal contamination. The operation was successfully completed. The patient was discharged after suture removal and the wound was healed well. The patient was walking with one leg and with the help of walking stick. After 3 months the patient came to me and demanded closure of colostomy. There was no anorectal Physiological laboratory in any centre in Tamil Nadu at that time. I did the indigenous way of testing the effective function of the rectum and anal canal by giving retention enema to assess the how much enema fluid he can hold and how long he has retained the enema fluid. The quantity of enema fluid was increased day to day. There was progress in the amount of fluid retaining power and the duration of retaining power. After 2 weeks the colostomy was closed. The patient was continent for a reasonable duration. The patient was in the ward for two weeks after colostomy closure to observe for faecal incontinence. He was a barber by profession. He never came for review to assess the continence.

27.4. LIPOMA NECK CARDIAC ARREST ON THE TABLE.

A case of lipoma in the neck posted for surgery as a op case. One house surgeon was operating and one PG was assisting him. When they gave field blocks and made the incision and preceding the surgery. The patient developed Cardiac arrest. Since the surgery was done under local, anaesthetist was not available by the side of the patient. I was informed about the Cardiac arrest; I immediately called the anaesthetist to pass the endotracheal tube and start O2 supplementation. I did the external Cardiac massage by Chest compression but heart beats was not restored. Then the anaesthetists said try Open Cardiac massage. So I did thoracotomy and gave open Cardiac massage. The heart beats regained but it was Cardiac fibrillation. By this time the chief anaesthetist came with defibrillator and applied it, after three applications the heart beats were restored and the peripheral pulse was palpable. The anaesthetist looked after further management and I closed the Chest wound. I was looking for the patient's relatives to inform the condition but nobody was available. I was worried because if death occurred how to inform the death to the relatives. We did not know the real name of the patient and place where he came and the address. I deputed one PG to be by the side of the patient to help the anaesthetist. When I came back at about 5 PM the patient was stable and I was told that one relative had come. I talked with him and asked him how he came to recovery room. He said the patient is his brother in law and the patient told him that it is only minor operation and will be back by 2 PM. Since he has not come by 3 PM I came to the operation theatre to enquire and I found him here. Now my mind was much relaxed. The patient was in the recovery room and died on the 5th day. I used to tell the students that no surgery is simple and no surgery is without complications.

27.5. PSUEDO CYST OF PANCREAS.

A 30 year old male had acute abdominal pain while he was working in the paddy field near Usilampatty. He was admitted as acute abdomen from casualty. On examination of the patient, acute pancreatitis was suspected. So along other blood investigations, serum Amylase estimation also requested. After 2 hours the Biochemistry lab technician phoned to the ward and asked about the case and what the suspected diagnosis is. I asked him have you estimated the serum Amylase and what is the value? He said, sir, it is more than thousand units; I have not seen such a high level. I told him that is what I wanted; it is a case of acute pancreatitis. I remember that prof. A.A.A., in theory class said the pain in acute pancreatitis will be so severe that if the patient lives next day it is acute pancreatitis, if he dies it is dissecting Aneurism and the serum Amylase level will be in four digits, it is a civil surgeon's pay. On those days the assistant surgeons pay was Rs.550 per month and the civil surgeon's pay was Rs.1000 per month. That is why he said like that four digits. The patient was treated conservatively.

He recovered well and discharged after 10 days. He was advised to come after 10 days. But he came only after 2 months with a epigastric cystic swelling, the psuedocyst of pancreas. It was confirmed by Ba.meal study. (No ultra sonogram at that time). He was posted for cysto gastrostomy. On the previous day of surgery during my night rounds I examined the patient; there was no mass in the epigastrium. It can happen in this condition. The fluid gets drained spontaneously due to internal drainage, when the obstruction of pancreatic duct (probably due to inflammatory obstruction) was relieved. The patient was discharged and he was reviewed after one month, there was no recurrence of the cyst.

27.6. BLOOD BANK AT VIRUDUNAGAR HOSPITAL.

Well established Blood Bank service was not available in1988-89 at Virudunagar hospital. My two predecessors referred major cases to

Madurai. For emergency cases in maternity, Blood grouping and cross matching and V.D.R.L test for the donor were done. There was one nurse who worked in Blood Bank in Chennai; I asked her help for blood collection from relative donors. I requested the D.M.O. to depute her service to Blood Bank in the morning duty. For those cases I feel blood may be required during surgery, I discuss with the patients relatives about the need for the blood. I told them, we will do blood test for those who are willing to donate blood and we will take blood only from the person whose blood is compatible to the patient. For the first case some people came forward to give blood and one person blood was compatible.

I asked that particular man to come to blood bank on the day of surgery at 9 AM after breakfast and wait there. If necessary we will take blood from you. He agreed to come at 9 AM. With the confident of availability of blood, I started the case and that patient did not required blood. Same thing has happened in other two cases. Now the relatives know that blood will be taken only when necessary. Many peoples volunteered to donate blood. So we have to do Blood grouping at least 4-5 persons for each patient. The Pharmacist told the D.M.O that we are using blood grouping sera about 5 times more than what we were using normally and there will be audit objection. D.M.O. asked me about this audit objection. I told, we are doing more cases and our operation statistic is 10 times more in general surgery. For all mayor cases we have to do blood grouping for the patients and also relative who were willing to donate and keep ready in case blood is required during surgery. If you want I will give it in writing now itself. The D.M.O. said because the pharmacist has objected for the large quantity of blood grouping sera where used for blood grouping I asked about it, now you have given the reason which I also agree. Then he called the pharmacist to indent more sera for blood grouping. There after there was no problem for blood grouping and cross matching. I did all mayor surgeries in Virudunagar hospital. But now the Blood Bank Law is enforced and I was told that Blood Bank services are available in all District head quarters Hospitals.

27.7. HODGKINS LYMPHOMA—CAME HERE TO DIE.

A 30 years male from Nagapattinam, astrologist by profession, came to our outpatient in G.R.H. with multiple cervical and axillary lymph nodes enlargements. Biopsy from the neck node was Hodgkin's lymphoma. He had chemotherapy with available drugs at that time. He responded well with the treatment for five courses. Every time he got admitted, had treatment and go to Nagapattinam. He was unmarried and there is nobody to look after him. Every time he was admitted I used to keep him in the ward 2-3 days more till he wanted discharge.

There was no response in the treatment when he got admitted on that particular visit. During rounds I told him that I am not satisfied with the progress in your condition. He said, I know I will not have any improvement this time but I have come here because at least so many people are here to look after me in the final stage where as in Nagapattinam nobody and I have come here to die. As he said, he died ten days after admission.

27.8. PERIPHERAL NEURECTOMY FOR INTRACTABLE PAIN IN TAO.

A patient was admitted in our unit for intractable pain in both legs due to Thrombo Angitis Oblitrans (TA0). The patient had bilateral Lumbar Sympathetctomy else were. He had Placenta implantation in GRH about 6 months back. I thought of referring the case to neurosurgery department for spinothalamic tract transaction. Before referring the case I discussed about this case with the neurosurgeon Dr.M.Natarajan. He asked me whether I have completed ward works and I said yes. He gave me a book from the department Library itself and asked me to read the topic on Peripheral Neurectomy in the department itself. After I read the topic he said first you do peripheral Neurectomy before you refer for spino thalamic tract Trans section. I also agreed to do Peripheral Neurectomy.

I explained the patient about the surgery and the Possibility of loss of sensation in the foot and even tropic ulcer formation because of loss of sensations. He agreed for the Surgery. Under local infiltration the anterior tibial nerve, Posterior tibial nerve, Peroneal nerve and the Sural nerves were identified and divided. There was marked improvement in the pain relief. Later I did two more cases will good result in the pain relief. I tried placenta implantation in some cases and I am not happy with the results.

27.9. HIDRADENITIS PROGRESSIVA.- MR.MOHIDEEN.

Mr. Mohideen was admitted for Hidradenitis progressiva in the gluteal region, with severe infection and foul smelling discharge. He was treated with antibiotics and repeated Curettage of the sinuses. There was no attendee by his side. To inform his relations that he is in G.R.H. Madurai for treatment, I put him on D.I.L (Dangerously ill List) and in formed the R.M.O. and the nursing Superintendent. Official letter was sent to the address given during admission by the R.M.O. In spite of that nobody has come to see him even other 15 days. He has given Kerala address. I asked Mohideen why nobody has come even after 15 days of our letter sent to the address given during admission. He said nobody will come and the address is a false one, because I do not have any body in Kerala.

Now I understand that he was an abandon person from his family because of the disease. I kept him in the ward for more than 3 months. As per the rule a patient cannot be kept in the ward for more than 3months. So for record purposes I discharged the patient after 85 days and readmitted him on the next day. One day I was making rounds in the morning Mohideen said ' I have an ambition". I asked him what it is. He said I want a dossai. I asked him one is enough or you want more. He said one is enough. I gave ten Rupees for two dossai to ward boy. Then one day he said if I die my body should be handed over to the Gorippalayam Darka. Though he was alright at that time, I promised that I will do that. After 10 days, his condition deterioted and told the nurse to inform me about the death. On that day at about 5 PM the nurse informed me that Mohideen died. I confirmed the death in person in the hospital and went to Gorippalayam Darka to inform. A retired nursing supervisor was there and I told him about the death of Mohideen. He said he will make arrangements to bring the body officially and we will do funeral according to our customs. I had so many cases that were treated by our team with some mental satisfaction and Mohideen was one among them. The satisfaction of treating a destitute for more than 3 months, fulfilled his ambition of eating dossai and arranged for funeral by his religious customs at Gorippalayam Darka. The purpose of life: Useful yourself and useful to others.

27.10. CARCINOMA OF OESOPHAGUS.

A patient from my native place came to Madurai for the treatment of dysphagia. Barium swallows suggestive of carcinoma oesophagus. I referred him to Cardio thoracic unit. After investigations they said surgery could not be done and advised irradiation. Because he has come from far away I kept him in our ward for irradiation. On the fifth day of irradiation, he developed Tracheo-oesophageal fistula which I noticed during my ward rounds in the morning. I discussed with the patient about the condition and explained the need for feeding gastrostomy. He said whatever you think you do it. I asked the nurse to prepare the case for feeding gastrostomy and told her I will be doing afterward works. After all the works are over I asked the nurse to send the case to the operation theatre. The nurse said the patient wants to talk to you. The patient said his daughter's marriage is to be within 2 days and tomorrow night is 'ponalaippu' function in my house. In our area (Tirunelveli) the marriage will be in bridegroom house and the bride will be taken in a procession in the morning of the marriage day. The patient said he will come to Madurai for surgery immediately after the marriage. If you can send me tomorrow morning for marriage you do surgery now. Otherwise I will go the village and come after marriage. I told him if I do surgery now you cannot go home tomorrow. So I will discharge you today itself and come after marriage. I advised him not to take any solid food, and take liquid in small quantity. I asked nurse to give 1.5 litres of I.V. fluids before he goes. He was very happy that I have discharged him. On the day of function in his house (on the previous night of marriage) some people compelled him to take the marriage function food. He just swallowed the solid food, and because of Tracheo oesophageal fistula, the food entered in to the respiratory tract and he died and the marriage was stopped. When my brother came to Madurai he told me that incidence. You will be strict in all cases but why you sent him to Mukkudal. If he was in the hospital, the marriage would have been held, and the couples would have come to Madurai to see him. His argument is also correct. I think my calculation in this case was wrong.

28. HONOUR IN MY PROFESSIONAL CAREER.

28.1. SENIOR GYNECOLOGIST SAW MY SURGERY DELORME.

From casualty I was transferred to Dr. Shanmugam unit. The other two assistants in that unit were my teachers. So I requested them to allow me to do duties all the admission days, SOT, and repeat op, for about two months. I told them that I may need their help when I face problems in the management of the cases. They agreed and said you can contact us at any time, and regularly one of us will come in the night to see the cases. One afternoon I got a memo to see a case in the Labour ward. As I was going to the Labour ward Dr.Logambal asked me where I am going. I told her I am on duty; I got a memo from Labour ward to see a case. She said ask some senior assistant to see the case. I told her I will see the case and inform them by phone about the findings and she left the place. I saw the case and there is no urgency in that case to get second opinion. Anyhow I informed Dr.Nagaian about the condition and he said he will see the case when he comes for the night rounds. In the night rounds he saw the case and advised to continue the same treatment which I have recommended.

After my return from UK, I started the colorectal unit in GRH. All the bottom cases were referred to colorectal op other than the surgical side. Dr.Logambal unit case will be brought by the PGs and they discuss with me about the case and I will give my opinion. Later all cases which require surgical opinion from her unit were sent to colorectal op which was conducted 3 days a week (on alternative days) between 10 and 12 noon. In these cases I will not write my opinion in the case sheet, the PGs will note down my findings and opinions in a separate paper to show it to her, because I am not supposed to see the general surgical cases other than the colorectal cases officially. I was doing one type perineal surgery (Delorme) for prolapsed rectum without opening the abdomen.

Dr. Logambal wanted to see that surgery. She asked my assistant whether he permit others to see his surgery. The assistant told her, he permits Doctors to see his surgery with permission, and I will inform you on the previous day about the time of surgery. When one patient was on bowel preparation for Delorme operation my assistant told me that Dr. Logambal is interested to see Delorme operation can I inform her to come to the theatre tomorrow. I said she was my teacher, I will be happy to see her in our theatre. The surgery went on more than one hour, throughout the surgery she was standing behind me to see to the operation where as I was sitting on a revolving stool while doing the surgery. I am honoured by the presence of my senior teacher and recognized me as a surgeon.

28.2. THREE CHILDREN WERE NAMED AFTER MINE.

In Watts and Johns orthopaedic text Book it is said usually the Obstetricians have the privilege that the children who were delivered by them, were named after the Obstetricians name but I had the privilege of three children named by my name.

A Government employee was treated by me for acid peptic disease some years back. He brought his daughter and son in law for investigations for sterility. I advised him to show his daughter to my wife Dr.Balasaraswathi and told him I will see your son in law.

After going through the history, I examined him. The vas difference on both sides had knot and the scar in the scrotum. I asked him confidently whether he had vasectomy previously. With some hesitation he accepted. Three years before marriage somebody forcefully had taken him for family planning surgery. I told him that it can be corrected by a minor surgery, I will not reveal to your wife and other family members. He agreed for the surgery. I told his wife and father in law that he needs a minor surgery to correct the defect and they also agreed. Vaso vasostomy was done on both sides. After one year she became pregnant and the delivery was conducted by my wife. At the time of discharge they said the child is named as Sivalingam.

Mr.Subbiah Nadar a patient from Thalavaipuram was operated 4th time for fistula by me. He was operated previously by some other surgeons. He had five daughters and no male child. At the time of fistula surgery, one of the daughters was pregnant. After some months my wife and me attended the marriage of his last daughter at Thirupparamkundrum after attending two marriages in Madurai and went to Thirupparamkundrum as last one.

We went to the marriage hall, they were preparing for vacating the marriage hall. The patient Mr. Subbiah Nadar called his daughter who was pregnant at the time of fistula surgery, and asked her to bring her recently delivered boy baby and asked her to tell the name of the child. She said the name as Sivalingam. Mr. Subbiah Nadar said doctor I am much impressed about your activities in the hospital and I have decided to name that child to be your name at that time itself.

A staff nurse working in colorectal op told me that she is going on leave for one month as she had planned to terminate her three months pregnancy. I asked her why she wanted to terminate the pregnancy. She said already I have two female children, if this is also female, it would be difficult to bring up three female children. At that time Scan was not available. I discussed with her that it may be a Male child so allow the pregnancy to continue, if this child is also female child and if you become pregnant again then you can go for Termination of pregnancy and sterilization or your husband can have vasectomy which I will do.

After discussing with her husband, they have decided to continue her pregnancy and if it is a Male child it will be named by my name. She delivered a boy baby. They were very happy, and thanked me for the advice. The nurse said the child's name is your name only.

ANNEXURE

I. PARTICULARS OF OPERATIONS DONE BY THE AUTHOR.

1974 to 1978.	Total cases.	838.
1983 to 1992.	Total cases.	3301.
1993 to 2002.	Total cases.	2899.
2003 to 2007.	Total cases.	1293.
2008 to 2o11.	Total cases.	619.
	Grand total	8950.
Per year number of cases		308.5.
Per month number of cases		26.

TOTAL COLORECTAL CASES.		(4252.)
1974 to 1978.	Total cases.	83.
1983 to 1992.	Total cases.	1948.
1993 to 2002.	Total cases.	1573.
2003 to 2007.	Total cases.	437.
2008 to 2011.	Total cases.	211.
	Grand total.	4252.

TOTAL GENERAL SURGERY CASES. (4698.)		
1974 to 1978.	Total cases.	755.
1983 to 1992.	Total cases.	1353.
1993 to 2003.	Total cases.	1326.

2003 to 2007. Total cases.   856.

2008 to 2011. Total cases.   408.

                 Grand total.   4698.

SOME IMPORTANT OPERATIONST IN COLORECTAL SURGERY.

1. Abdominoperineal Resection.   209.
2. Anterior Resection   61.
3. Right hemi Colectomy   40.
4. Left hemi Colectomy   13.
5. Ca.Rectum. Local excision   13.
6. Adenoma Rectum excision   8.
7. Polyps Rectum excision   65.
8. Total Colectomy   8.
9. Roscoe Graham operation   24.
10. Delorme operation   117.
11. Colostomy   88.
12. Colostomy Refashioning   27.
13. Colostomy closure   28.
14. Parastomal hernia   2.
15. Ileo transverse colostomy   11.
16. Ileo pelvic anatomises   6.
17. Subtotal Colectomy   12.
18. Faecal fistula   9.
19. Recto vaginal fistula   8.
20. Recto urethral fistula   1.
21. Swenson operation   6.
22. Gastrojejunocolic fistula   2.
23. Appendicectomy   157.

24. Anal sphincter repair	57.
25. Ca. Anal canal. Local excision.	8.
26. Piles	881.
27. Fistula	1173.
28. Fissure in ano	769.
29. Pilonidal sinus	40.
30. Anal warts	88.

IMPORTENT OPERATIONS IN GENERAL SURGERY.

1. Prostate	18.
2. Orchedectomy	7.
3. Hydrocele	105.
3. Vaso vasostomy	13.
4. Nephrectomy	5.
5. Urethral dilation	69.
6. Cholecystectomy	85.
7. Common Bile duct Strictures	6.
8. Posterior gastrojejunostomy	244.
9. Highly selective Vagotomy	21.
10. Gastrectomy	29.
11. Duodenal Perforation	39.
12. Feeding gastrostomy	8.
13. Tanners operation	13.
14. Splenectomy	12.
15. Laparotomy	47.
16. Inguinal hernia	467.
17. Incisional hernia	123.
18. Umbilical hernia	71.

19. Secondary Suturing	19.
20. Thyroid	81.
21. Lymph node biopsy	153.
22. Parotid gland	25.
23. Mastectomy	25.
24. Fibro adenoma Breast	132.
25. Intestinal obstructed	32.
26. Pancreatico- Jejunostomy.	6.
27. Lumbar sympathetctomy	9.
28. Varicose veins	22.
29. Peritoneo venous Shunt	12.
30. Skin grafting	11.
31. Tracheostomy	4.
32. Peripheral Neurectomy	3.
33. Thoracic duct internal Jugular vein anatomises.	5.

II. LIST OF PUBLICATIONS.

1. Uterus in inguinal hernia in a"Male". Indian Medical Gazette. 1977.
2. Surgical emergency. Antiseptic. 1997.
3. Mortality in general surgical practice. The Indian Practitioner.1979.
4. Specific Granulomatous lesions of the intestine. Indian Medical Gazette.1979.
5. Acute Retention of Urine. Antiseptic.1980.
6. Fibroangioma of Jejunum. Antiseptic 1980.
7. Irritable bowel syndrome. Antiseptic G.I.D. Special.1980.
8. Laparotomy, Delights and Disappointments. Indian Medical Gazette 1981.
9. Emergency Surgery for Inflammatory Catastrophes. Antiseptic. 1981.

10. Hepatomegaly in Surgical Practice. The Indian Practitioner. 1981.

11. Tracheostomy. Indications and complications. Antiseptic. 1981.

12. A critical study on colorectal cancer. Indian Medical Gazette. 1981.

13. Jejuno Gastric Intussusceptions. Indian Journal of Surgery. 1982.

14. Pattern of Abdominal Injury in Southern part of Tamil Nadu. Indian Journal Surgery 1982.

15. A Study on Amputation. The Indian Practitioner.1985.

16. A Rare Complication of Meckel's Diverticulam. The Indian Practitioner. 1985.

17. Hydatid Disease in a Teaching Hospital. Indian Journal of surgery. 1985.

18. Anterior Cervical Chemodectoma. Antiseptic 1985.

19. Peritoneo Venous Shunt for Intractable Ascites. Current Medical Trends. 1986.

20. Meckel's Diverticulam Clinical presentation. Indian Journal of surgery. 1987.

21. Gastroentrogy in Diabetes. Indian medical Association. Tamil Nadu 1989.

22. External duodenal fistula. Journal of Indian Medical Association. 1989.

23. Trans anal Surgical Procedure for Complete Rectal Prolapse. Digestive surgery Colon and Rectum. 1988.

24. Complete Prolapsed Rectum Treated by Trans Anal Surgical Technique. Experience with 98 cases. Indian Journal of Coloproctolgy.2001.

25. Best Approach for Management of Rectal Prolapse. Bombay Hospital Journal 2008.

III. PAPER PRESENTED IN VARIOUS CONFERENCES.

1. Blunt Injury Abdomen.
2. 1000 Cases of Gastroduodinal Surgery.

3. Colorectal Tumours.
4. External Abdominal Hernias.
5. Per operative Peritoneal Lavage.
6. Trans Anal Surgical technique for Prolapsed Rectum.(Singapore)
7. Tuberculosis of Colon.
8. Is there any Changing Patterns in Clinical Presentation of Peptic ulcer within a Decade? (Japan)
9. Management of Colostomy.
10. Piles A Profile of its Management.
11. Delorme Operation. (Sandeogo. USA)
12. Public Utility Service of Colorectal Surgery.
13. A Rare Complication Following Fistula surgery.
14. Intestinal Polyposis.
15. Multiple Polyposis coli.
16. Prevalence of Fistula in Ano in Madurai.
17. Sigmoidoscopy Evaluation. Twelve years Experience
18. Pilonidal sinus.
19. Infrared Coagulation in Treatment of Piles.
20. Papillary Medullary Carcinoma Thyroid.
21. Non traumatic Small bowel Lesions.
22. Pseudo Endemic Intussusceptions Is it Reality?.
23. Diagnostic Laparoscopy in General Surgery.
24. One hundred Cases of Thyroid Surgery.
25. Sigmoidoscopy its value in Chronic Diarrhoea.
26. Adult Hirschsprung's Disease.

IV. LECTURES GIVEN IN CME, CONFERENCES, AND IMA.

Lectures were given in different places in CME, Conferences of various Associations in surgery and Indian Medical Association in Tamil Nadu. Total lectures of 92 Topics were given.

V. WORKSHOPS.

Conducted Five Workshops in Madurai. Faculty member in Five Workshops in different parts of India.

DISTINCTION AND AWARDS:

1. Common wealth Medical Fellowship Award in Colorectal Surgery in 1981-82 Sessions. Had training in The General Infirmary Leeds and St Marks hospital London, UK.
2. Governing Council Member of The Tamil Nadu Dr.M.G.R. Medical University (Governor Nominee) from August 2000 for 3 years.
3. Director of Surgical studies in Association of Surgeons of India for 3 years 2001-2003.
4. Chairman of Tamil Nadu and Pondicherry Chapter of ASI in 1998.
5. President of Association of Colon and Rectal Surgeons India for two years 1995- 96.
6. President Ostomates India Madurai chapter from 1994 to 2015.
7. Examiner for Fellowship in Colon and Rectal Surgeons of India from 2001 to 2011.
8. Chairman board of Examination of ACRSI 2008 to 2011.
9. Member of Academic Committee Medical Council of India New Delhi to start Mch in Colorectal Surgery.
10. Examiner in Surgery for both under graduates and post graduates in various Universities in southern part of India.
11. Life time Achievement Award received from:

    i. Asian federation of Coloprctology. (2009)

    ii. Association of Colon and Rectal Surgeons of India. (2009).

    iii. The Tamil Nadu Dr. M.G.R Medical university.(2012).
12. Honorary fellow in:

    i. Fellow of the Association of Surgeons of India (1993)

    ii. Fellow of Association of Colon and Rectal Surgeons of India.1999

    iii. Fellow of International Society of Colopractoloy.2014.

BOOK AUTHOR /EDITOR/CONTRIBUTION:

1. C.M.E. Proceedings WVIII conference of Tamil Nadu and Pondicherry Chapter of ASI (1993) Tirunelveli. Chapter of Carcinoma of Anal Region.

2. Recent Advances in Surgery 6. By Roshanlal Gupta 1998. Chapter on Complete Rectal Prolepses A personal experience.

3. Basic sciences in Colo Proctology1999 Editor. Publisher Ezhil Madurai. Chapter on Fistula in Ano.

4. Recent Advances in Surgery 7. By Roshanlal Gupta 2000. Chapter on Colonic Pseudo Obstruction.

5. Progress in Surgery LXI ASICON 2001. Edited by A. Khandelwal. Chapter on Colostomy Care.

6. Progress in Surgery LXII ASICON 2002. Edited by Asit KR.Banerjee. Chapter on Necrotizing Fasciitis.

7. Book on Topic in Colorectal Surgery. Japee Brothers Medical Publications (P) LTD 2010.

8. Benign Anorectal Disorders. Published by Springer. December 2015. Two Chapters I. Haemorrhoids. II. Pelvic Floor Dysfunction.

9. Enname Vazhvu. A book on Ostomy in Tamil 2002.

10. Kanavukalum Nikalvukalum.(Tamil) Published by Srinivasa Fine Arts (P) LTD. Sivakasi 2017.

11. Marakka Eyalatha Payana Anubavangal.(Tamil) Manivasagar Pathippagam. Chennai. 2018.

www.ingramcontent.com/pod-product-compliance
Lightning Source LLC
Chambersburg PA
CBHW030757180526
45163CB00003B/1065